SALPÊTRIÈRE

SALPÊTRIÈRE
The Story of a Hospital

*From Tyranny and Horror
to Caring and Renown*

Doug Addy

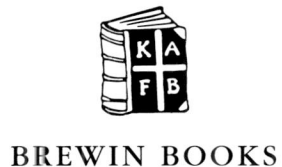

BREWIN BOOKS

BREWIN BOOKS
19 Enfield Ind. Estate,
Redditch,
Worcestershire,
B97 6BY
www.brewinbooks.com

Published by Brewin Books 2022

© Douglas Addy 2022

The author has asserted his rights in accordance with the Copyright, Designs and Patents Act 1988 to be identified as the author of this work.

All rights reserved. No part of this publication may be reproduced, stored in a retrieval system, or transmitted in any form or by any means, electronic, mechanical, photocopying, recording or otherwise, without the prior permission in writing of the publisher and the copyright owners, or as expressly permitted by law, or under terms agreed with the appropriate reprographics rights organization. Enquiries concerning reproduction outside the terms stated here should be sent to the publishers at the UK address printed on this page.

The publisher makes no representation, express or implied, with regard to the accuracy of the information contained in this book and cannot accept any legal responsibility for any errors or omissions that may be made.

Front cover image (top): Salpêtrière Hospital.
© Mbzt (CC-BY-SA/3.0).

A CIP catalogue record for this book is available from the British Library.

ISBN: 978-1-85858-750-9

Printed and bound in Great Britain
by 4edge Ltd.

Contents

Acknowledgements   viii

Preface   ix

Introduction   xi

Part 1 – The Salpêtrière Hospital

Chapter 1 – The Sun King   2
Louis XIV, Cardinal Mazarin, St. Vincent de Paul

Chapter 2 – Nightfall   8
The little arsenal, the new hospital, the detainment centre, stories of the French Colonies

Chapter 3 – Nightmare   12
Revolution, Massacre

Chapter 4 – A New Dawn   17
Pinel, Esquirol, Duchenne

Chapter 5 – Daybreak   28
Charcot, Bottard

Chapter 6 – The Charcot School   43
Bourneville, Charcot's famous son (Jean Baptiste Charcot), Gilles de la Tourette, Bouchard, Babinski

Chapter 7 – After Charcot   61
Brissaud, Raymond, Dejerine, Klumpke (Madame Dejerine)

Chapter 8 – Perpetuating the Fame   65
Marie, Guillain, Barré, Aicardi

Part 2 – Beyond the Salpêtrière

Chapter 9 – Charcot's Contemporaries in Neurology   74
*Brown-Séquard, Broca, Hughlings Jackson, Quincke,
Gowers, Ramón y Cajal, Horsley, Alzheimer, Cushing*

Chapter 10 – Charcot's Contemporaries in Biological Science   90
Bernard, Pasteur, Sherrington

Part 3 – The Background

France in the Time of Charcot   98

Chapter 11 – The Bourbon Restoration (1814-1830)   100
*Louis XVIII, Charles X, Louis Philippe
President Louis Napoleon/Emperor Napoleon III*

Chapter 12 – The Paris Commune of 1871   105
Thiers, Clemenceau

Chapter 13 – The Belle Époque (1871-1914)   108
*The engineers, the artists, the musicians,
the cabaret, the novelists, Zola, Dreyfus*

Epilogue   118

Bibliography   119

Index   121

Dedication

To my parents Edmund (Ted) and Ivy Irene Pauline (Reenie) whose devotion, along with a grant from Barnsley Town Council, made it possible for a boy from the backstreets of the south Yorkshire coalfield to have a life and a career that his ancestors could never have dreamed of. To my wife Jennifer, who stood by my side and was my anchor for nigh on 50 years and to Richard, Kate, Chris, Jess and our grandsons George and Joe, whom Jennifer never met.

* * * *

In memory of my wife and of two close friends, all royalties from the sale of this book will be divided equally between Cancer Research UK and Alzheimer's Research UK.

Acknowledgements

I thank (in no particular order); my friends Arthur and Barbara Gennard and Mike and Barbara Colclough whose comments changed the nature of the book; my friend and fellow paediatrician Martin Brueton for examining the text and for his kind comments; my friend John Bastable for computer help, my daughter Kate for her enthusiasm and encouragement; my neighbour Ruth McCormack for help when needed and Alistair Brewin and his staff for their expert supervision of gestation and delivery.

Preface

I am a long-retired general paediatrician with a particular interest in paediatric neurology. I spent my consultant career at City Hospital Birmingham (Dudley Road Hospital when I was first appointed), a large general hospital in one of the more deprived areas of Birmingham. During this terrible pandemic I have often found myself in virtual solitary confinement, living alone as a widower and at high risk as an 81 year old with chronic chest disease (bronchiectasis as a result of whooping cough as a baby). For physical exercise I have an exercise bike and in the attempt to prevent my brain turning to jelly I turn to writing. It has always been my main hobby; I have written many articles in the medical journals. But what to write about?

Many years ago, when I was a senior registrar at the Alder Hey Children's Hospital in Liverpool, I saw a child in the paediatric neurology clinic of Dr. John Roberts. I noticed that the child had muscle wasting of the lower parts of the legs (so-called 'inverted champagne bottle legs') characteristic of Charcot-Marie-Tooth disease. That set me wondering about these people Charcot, Marie and Tooth. I discovered that Charcot and Marie had worked in Paris during the 19th century at a hospital with the intriguing name of La Salpêtrière (the saltpetre 'gunpowder' factory hospital). At the same time Tooth was an English physician at Saint Bartholomew's and the Queen Square Nervous Diseases hospitals in London. In Liverpool my clinical duties meant that I was unable to look into it any further but I always retained at the back of my mind the thought of pursuing it again sometime.

Like many people and famously like Cole Porter, I love Paris. I first visited that vibrant, romantic city with my wife Jennifer on our honeymoon and we returned several times, including on our Ruby Wedding Anniversary (we got to within five months of Gold when we would probably have made it again). I hope to return once more when this pestilence is gone, to see the magnificent 17th century buildings still standing alongside the buildings of the modern hospital. And so, here was the opportunity and this book is the result.

I have tried to present as accurate an account as possible with the resources available to me. If there are inaccuracies, they are the result of my own misconceptions allied to the vagaries of historical reporting: what Lucy Worsley would call 'the fibs of history'.

Doug Addy
Henley in Arden
July 2022

Introduction

Some names have a mysterious magic that acts in the way of a skilfully thrown lasso to draw us in like wandering steers. Think of Ishmael, think of Manderley, think of Timbuktu or Katmandu, with its one-eyed yellow idol to the north that Kipling, apparently, didn't write about. I knew a man in Katmandu… now there's an opening line to rival Melville or Du Maurier, all it needs is a book to follow it. That's the trouble with first lines, you can have it for free.

Dharma Manandhar, later professor of paediatrics in Katmandu, was the registrar in paediatrics when I arrived at Dudley Road Hospital as a newly appointed consultant in 1972. We were friends for years. We visited him and his family in Katmandu and I spoke to his students. Ever cheerful and smiling with an infectious chuckle he is a delightful man, he could have had a successful career in paediatrics in the UK with greater financial reward but less in terms of reward of the heart. He chose to return home to serve the people of his own country and he made fundamental and much applauded advances in the care of mothers and babies in rural Nepal and similar impoverished and isolated places around the world. We lost touch, I don't know quite how, but I hope he is well and thriving. I read that he is now the head of an NGO that promotes the care of such mothers and babies, he is 'a better man than I am' and that *is* Kipling. George Orwell once described W H Auden as "a sort of gutless Kipling", I don't know how Auden upset him but it seems that he may have agreed, I learn from a recent issue of *The Week* that he agreed to have some of his poems included in an anthology only with the addition of a note explaining that he thought they were trash and was ashamed he had written them.

This is the story of a hospital called Salpêtrière (well, if London can have its Arsenal why shouldn't Paris have its Salpêtrière?). I think it was the name that first caught me, but the more I looked into it the tighter became the rope until it became so tight that I had to tell you about it.

"It may seem a very strange principle to enunciate as the very first requirement of a hospital that it should do the sick no harm."
       Florence Nightingale. *Notes on hospitals,* 1863 (Preface).

In fact, it wasn't all that strange, because Hippocrates of Kos had got in, as regards doctors, with the same principle, *primum non nocere,* 'first do no harm' just a couple of thousand years before. Even that has a connection to this story because Auguste François Chomel (1788-1858), a Parisian physician and successor to Laennec as Professor of Clinical Medicine at the Paris Faculty, is said to have brought the phrase *primum non nocere* into modern medical awareness.

It is a truth to be considered appropriate (and a source of pride without prejudice) that many of the great hospitals of the world are in the relatively deprived areas of big cities. Such a hospital is the Salpêtrière Hospital in the 13th arrondissement of Paris, on the left bank of the Seine, just to the east of the Latin Quarter and within easy walking distance of Notre-Dame. The story begins with King Louis XIV of France.

Part 1

The Salpêtrière Hospital

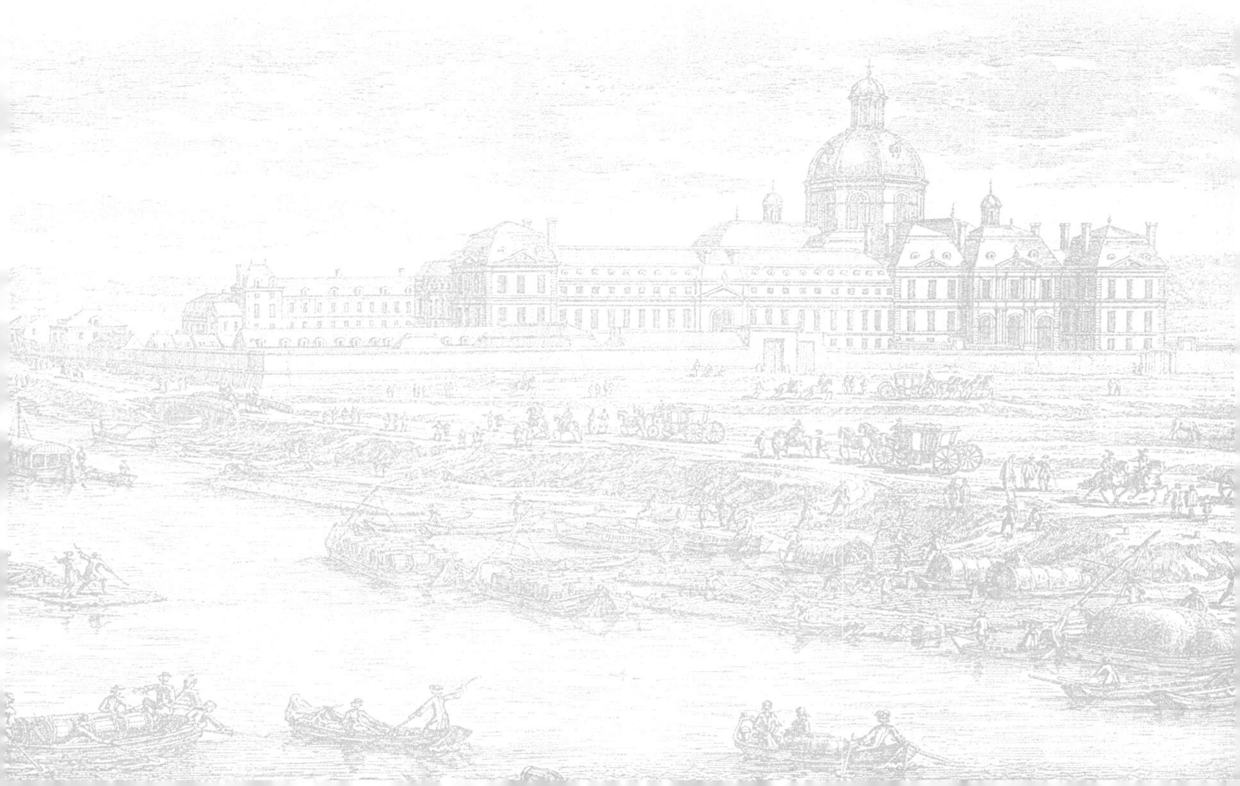

Chapter 1

The Sun King

"Despotism is unjust to everybody, including the despot, who probably was made for better things."
                    Oscar Wilde, *The Soul of Man Under Socialism* (Essay) 1891.

"Tyranny: a deviant form of kingship."
                              Attributed to Aristotle (384-322 BC).

Louis XIV (1638-1715)

Louis XIV of the house of Bourbon was born at 11.22am on Sunday the 5th of September 1638 in the chateau of Saint Germain-en-Laye, a royal palace in the department of Yvelines some 12 miles west of Paris. His mother was Anne of Austria and his ostensible father was Louis XIII but he probably wasn't the biological father. Louis XIII was reportedly gay and there is doubt (but not much) about the consummation of the marriage; he had certainly not visited his wife's bed for many years before the birth. Several real fathers have been proposed but by far the most likely is Cardinal Mazarin. Anne had suffered a series of miscarriages and was just short of 37 when the child was born so the birth was regarded as miraculous and the baby a gift of god, which led to him being named Louis Dieudonné.

   Young Louis became King in 1643 on the death of Louis XIII when he was four years and seven months old. Anne was declared Regent two days later but the power behind the throne was Cardinal Mazarin whom Anne quickly appointed as chief minister. Although Louis was said to have reached his majority by the age of 13, he did not assume the reins of power until Mazarin died in 1661 when Louis was 22. Mazarin had been a father to Louis and a life partner to Anne (see later). From then on Louis guarded his absolute power with absolute determination.

1. The Sun King

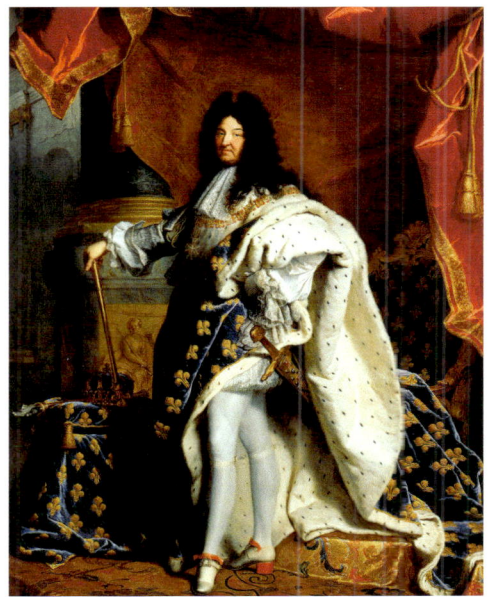
Louis XIV.

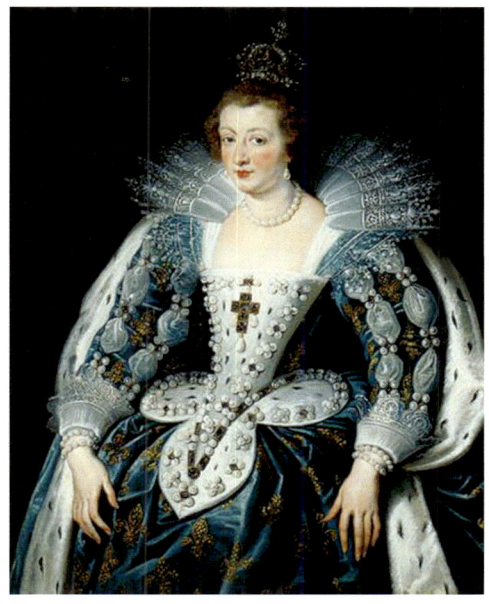
Anne of Austin.

He was King for 72 years and 110 days, a record for European monarchy, although Elizabeth II is catching up (70 years at the time of writing). During his reign he fought four major wars and many smaller wars and skirmishes including the War of Devolution (1667-68), the Dutch War (1672-78), the War of the League of Augsberg (1688-97) and the War of the Spanish Succession (1702-13). Clearly he was not usually one to end a scrap in a hurry. He acquired the titles of 'Louis the Great' and 'the Sun King' while presiding over monstrous tyranny, but was credited with having added greatly to the glory of France. He died on Sunday the 1st of September 1715 with gangrene of his left leg.

Was Louis a cruel man? Anthony Levi hesitates to say it but believes he was *quite* cruel, his answer to the question is a Delphic 'more yes than no'. Perhaps biographers tend to develop an attachment to their biographees, a sort of biographers' Stockholm syndrome. Levi describes Louis as a bully, ascribing it to his unrestricted power and a basic feeling of insecurity. But doesn't all bullying stem from power and the need to show it and isn't all bullying cruel? The powerful need not be bullies. As we shall see, it seems unlikely that the women being dragged against their will into the Salpêtrière, or cowering with fright in a small wooden ship on the high seas of the Atlantic not knowing their fate, would have hesitated.

Between 1648 and 1653 France suffered a series of two civil wars called the Fronde. As with that other, transatlantic, war of 1775-1783 the issue was taxation. A major result of the Fronde was a very great and lamentable increase in poverty and begging. The authorities really didn't know what to do about the beggars but they 'defiled' the streets of Paris so they confined them, providing little or no medical care but ridding the streets of the 'riffraff' (Riffraff: worthless people, from Old French *rif et raf* related to *rifler* to plunder and *rafle* a sweeping up. It's a harsh and abhorrent word but in this context strangely apt).

There is an arched entrance to the hospital above which stand the names of four men, Cardinal Mazarin, St. Vincent de Paul, Philippe Pinel and Jean-Martin Charcot. Pinel and Charcot are main participants in this story and will appear in due course. For now I shall refer to the first two of the four.

Cardinal Mazarin (1601-1661)

Cardinal father of a King; statesman, teacher; everything.

Mazarin was born into an Italian upper class family. He attended the Jesuit College in Rome from the age of seven and from the age of 20 he studied law at the University of Madrid. As a teenager he indulged in gambling, usually losing, and in 1628 he obtained a doctorate in law in Rome. Later that year he was taken on as a secretary by a papal diplomat and it was then that he met Cardinal Richelieu, Louis XIII's chief minister of malign repute (wasn't he the French equivalent of Robin Hood's Sheriff of Nottingham?). At least, that's what I learned from the *Three Musketeers* films as a child. He was always introduced by a brief clash of sinister music, like when the Indians appeared in cowboy films. Mazarin impressed Richelieu, although they didn't always see eye to eye, and the senior man had him made cardinal in 1638 though he was

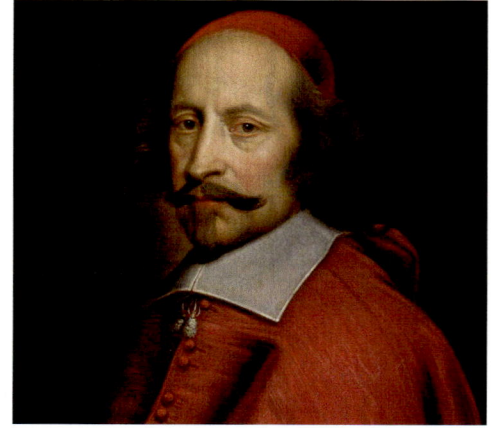

Cardinal Mazarin.

never a priest. On the deaths of Richelieu in 1642 and Louis XIII five months later in 1643, he became chief minister to Queen Anne, when she was made Regent to the child Louis XIV two days after she became a widow. By that time Mazarin had been working at the French court for some time and it is popularly believed that he was the father of the young King. Some historians believe Mazarin and Anne were secretly married, others do not. Cardinals, of course, are not allowed to marry nor to have children: neither, I suppose, are Queens entitled to marry in secret. But they were both probably fairly well versed in the arts of intrigue and secrecy; Mazarin certainly had a Machiavellian side to his nature. From the time he was appointed chief minister, he devoted himself to the education of the child King and to running the affairs of France involving many wars, mainly against Spain, and the two-part civil war of the Fronde.

The two parts of the Fronde were the parliamentary Fronde of 1648-9 and the Fronde of the Princes of 1650-53 (a *fronde* is a catapult such as may be used by children or by rebels on the street). The first Fronde was the result of excessive taxation which was resisted by the nobles who formed the parliament, a purely advisory body. Mazarin had the parliamentary leaders arrested and a general rebellion burst onto the streets. A peace was negotiated in 1649.

The second Fronde involved Princes and military leaders in a struggle for power and opposition to Mazarin. Eventually the rebellious Princes were defeated leaving the field open to absolute rule by Louis XIV. The effect of all this on the national finances was dramatic, leading to widespread poverty and a very marked increase in the number of beggars. This in turn led to the clearing of the beggars from the streets and to the establishment of the *Hôpital Général de Paris* and the Salpêtrière in which Mazarin played a large part, some of it charitable and some not.

St. Vincent de Paul (1581-1660)

"With malice toward none; with charity for all."
Abraham Lincoln, *2nd Inaugural Address*, 1865.

Vincent de Paul is known as the patron saint of charity or charities. He was born into a family of peasant farmers in the small village of Pouy, in the department of Landes in what is now Nouvelle Aquitaine in west and southwest France. Since 1828 the village has taken the name of St. Vincent de Paul.

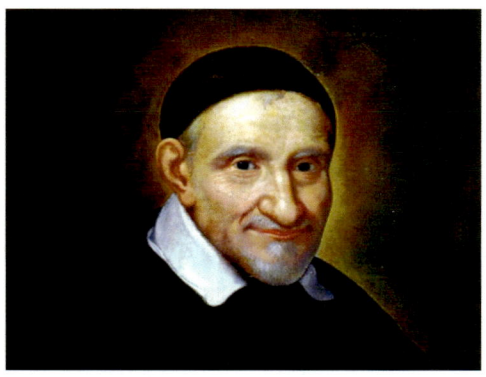
St. Vincent de Paul.

After an impoverished country childhood he entered a seminary at the age of 15. He studied theology at the University of Toulouse and was ordained in 1600, when he was 19. There is considerable debate about his time as a young priest, his letters suggest that he was taken prisoner by Barbary pirates and enslaved but this account is not believed by many historians; they presumably believe that the future saint lied. Whatever the truth he seems to have had a succession of 'masters' one of whom was a practitioner of spagyric medicine, a form of alchemy. He eventually worked his way back to France and then Rome. By 1612 he was a parish priest in Clichy near Paris and there he began his association with the Daughters of Charity an organisation of women within the church. In 1622 he acted as chaplain to the galley slaves in Paris and began to run the Congregation of the Mission whose aim was to provide relief to the poor. He was instrumental in organising retreats and seminaries for the education of the priesthood, who at that time were on the whole, a quite ignorant and impious set of people (he had, himself, initially entered the Church with the idea of a quiet and easy life.) In 1643, that momentous year in the history of the Bourbons, he became spiritual adviser to Queen Anne. It was perhaps his influence on Anne, and by extension on Mazarin and Louis XIV, that brought such charity as there was to the establishment of the General Hospital and the Salpêtrière. He was canonised in 1737.

The new hospital

From explosives to correctives, but seldom curatives.

Originally, the main Paris arsenal was on the right bank of the river but the people complained about the danger, there having been an occasional explosion, and Louis was persuaded to build a 'Little Arsenal' on the left bank at a place outside the city limits. Gunpowder is 75% saltpetre (potassium nitrate), 15% charcoal and 10% sulphur, so the little arsenal became known as the saltpetre factory, in French 'La Salpêtrière'. Beset with the Fronde, Vincent de Paul organised the charities, the President of Parliament, Pomponne de Bellièvre,

1. The Sun King

persuaded Mazarin to provide the buildings of the Little Arsenal, and the complex of the *Hôpital Général de Paris* was formed, the main components of which were the Bicêtre, the Pitié, and the Salpêtrière. In 1656 Louis issued an edict establishing the General Hospital and all the beggars on the streets of Paris were arrested.

The Salpêtrière Hospital was built between 1657 and 1669 and was used to confine prostitutes and other women considered undesirable and there was, in effect, a small village for mainly elderly and infirm women. In 1680 the Prison de la Force was built for 'riotous beggars' and in 1684 the King extended the remit to "prostitutes, debauched girls incapable of reform, prisoners of the king, and women guilty of adultery". Later, one part of the building carried the name of Benjamin Franklin and there was an open court with a fountain which was still there in Guillain's time (1920s to 50s, he will appear) and by which it was fondly believed the fictional Manon Lescaut had taken her rest periods. Further alterations to the buildings were done in the 18th century but the old buildings are now preserved alongside the modern hospital buildings.

The new Salpêtrière Hospital was a grand affair quite befitting the King who was to build and occupy the palace of Versailles. The architect was Libéral Bruant who had designed the Hôtel des Invalides, which now houses the tomb of Napoleon, and was a man of great reputation. But it wasn't a hospital the likes of which you and I have ever known.

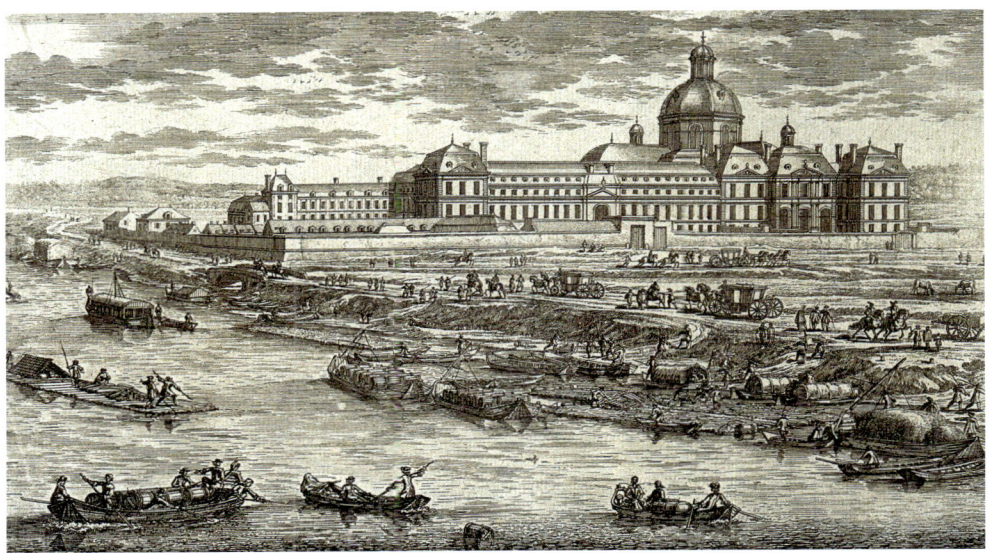

The building of the Salpêtriere.

Chapter 2

Nightfall

"The long dark night of tyranny."
                    Ed Murrow, American journalist. Broadcast 1954.

Detainment centre

One class of women overrepresented at the Salpêtrière were the prostitutes. The plan being to remove the 'riffraff' from the streets of Paris, the many prostitutes of the city were rounded up and carted off to the dismal depths of what was by now the despised, rat-ridden hellhole they called 'La Salpêtrière'. It was a place for women only; the equivalent men's hospital was the Bicêtre three miles away and the women in the Salpêtrière would often be paired off with men from the Bicêtre and shipped off to populate the French colonies of the New World. Some would be sent individually and auctioned off on arrival with a marriage ceremony the following day (the Bicêtre is named after the Kremlin Bicêtre, a suburban commune in southern Paris. Kremlin in this case probably comes from an ancient Greek word meaning citadel. There is a station on the Paris metro called Kremlin Bicêtre).

One of those women was the heroine of the Antoine Prévost novel and Puccini opera, *Manon Lescaut*. She was a courtesan who, for the crime of prostitution, was imprisoned in the Salpêtrière, finished up in Louisiana and died in the malaria-infested swamps of the lower Mississippi delta. Of course, it's a myth, there was no Manon Lescaut. But there were many

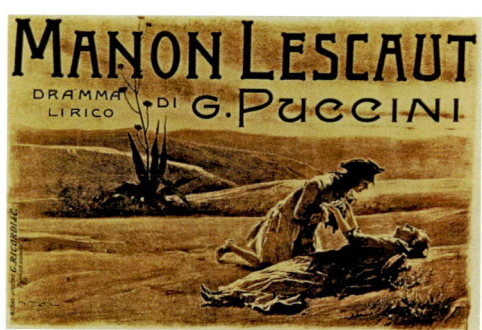

Puccini's opera.

2. Nightfall

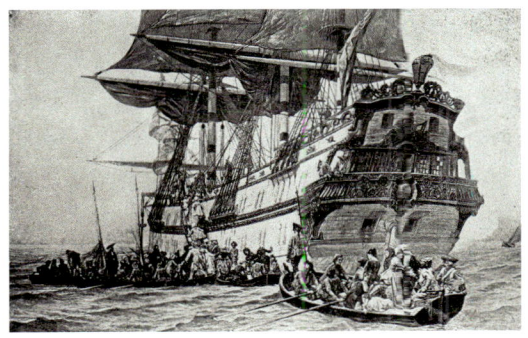

Embarkation of Manon Lescaut.

Manon Lescauts and Louis could think of nastier punishments; apparently he ordered that any prostitute found with one of his soldiers within five miles of the palace was to forfeit her nose and ears. Perhaps he had a giant compass to draw a circle to demonstrate the extent of the prohibition. It seems not so much that he objected to what they did but that he objected to them doing it under his nose. That's why he had all those people removed from the streets of Paris; they got under, or up, his nose. Whether such a punishment was ever carried out I don't know. It seems hardly likely the man was going to report it (unless he thought he was not getting value for money), but I suppose they might have been caught *in flagrante*. The police would have had to have looked pretty hard though. He wasn't really a cruel man, of course, he did it out of kindness. The embarkation of Manon Lescaut for Louisiana is portrayed in the 1883 painting by Charles Édouard Delort *L'embarquement de Manon Lescaut.*

Another long term involuntary resident of the Salpêtrière, this time indisputably non-fictional, was Anne-Josèphe Théroigne de Méricourt. Born in 1762 in Marcourt in the prince-bishopric of Liege in Belgium, she became active and prominent in the French Revolution and was noted for her great beauty but because of the rampant sexism of the time she was ridiculed and dismissed by the anti-revolutionary press. As a revolutionary she was captured, imprisoned and interrogated in Austria. On her release she returned to Paris and was lauded as a hero of the revolution but her fervour turned to

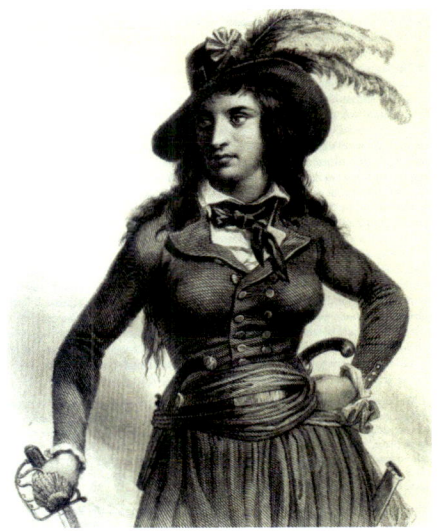

Anne-Josèphe Théroigne de Méricourt.

madness. She was obsessed with the revolution and would speak constantly and of nothing else. One doctor offered a diagnosis of 'revolutionary fever' but Esquirol, a prominent psychiatrist at the Salpêtrière (see later), later diagnosed manic depression, which I suppose is another way of saying bipolar disease. She was passed from asylum to asylum before spending the last 10 years of her life (1807-17) confined within the Salpêtrière. Simon Schama looks upon her as a prototype of Marianne, the symbol throughout France of the revolutionary origins of the republic, portrayed in the famous 1830 painting by Delacroix *Liberty leading the people*, the subject of which is the 1830 revolution when King Charles X was deposed and replaced by King Louis Philippe, though the painting is often used as an illustration of the first revolution of 1789-1799, what most people mean when they refer to 'The French Revolution'.

Stories of the French Colonies, True and Untrue

Les filles du roi

Many women at the Salpêtrière were forcefully deported but some chosen women, deemed to be less culpable, were allowed to volunteer and presumably treated better. The colonists began to complain about the poor quality of arrivals from France and Louis supported a plan to encourage young women of attested character to move to New France in Canada with financial inducements. They were called 'les filles du roi' and more than 830 took up the offer in the 10 years after 1663. Some were 'returned to seller' as not being of 'saleable quality' because of either a lack of moral character, or insufficient hardiness to withstand the Canadian winters. The descendants of the filles du roi are said to include Hillary Clinton, Angelina Jolie and Madonna.

The Brides of la Baleine

On 8th January 1721 the French ship *Baleine* arrived off the coast of Mississippi. Its passengers included a group of around 80 young women who had been approved by the Cardinal Archbishop of Paris as of sufficient rectitude to leave the village of the Salpêtrière and emigrate to the French colony based in Louisiana. The group settled successfully in Biloxi, Mississippi, not far from New Orleans, and is now looked upon along the Gulf Coast with the same reverence as is given in the rest of America to the Plymouth Colony in

Massachusetts. The *Baleine* is said to have contributed almost as many genes to the American genepool as did the *Mayflower*. The Brides of la Baleine is an organisation similar to the Daughters of the Mayflower.

The Casquette Girls (Les Files à la cassette)

The Casquette Girls were named so after the small chests (casquettes) in which they transported their clothes. They came from convents and religious orphanages with a guarantee of virginity and were sent to the Canadian French colonies, Louisiana and the West Indies. Or so it was said. Recent historians, however, have kiboshed the whole business claiming that there were no such people as the casquette girls; it was all a myth. The fibs of history again, just as I was imagining the crinolinned young women trotting off the ships, their suitcases in hand, hoping against hope to find happiness in a foreign clime and closing my eyes and hoping that they did. I have now learned that crinolines did not appear until the mid-19th century and the similar dress in the 17th century was the farthingale.

Chapter 3

Nightmare

"In the nightmare of the dark, all the dogs of Europe bark."
WH Auden, In memory of WB Yeats, 1940.

Revolution

"Those who make peaceful revolution impossible will make violent revolution inevitable."
President John F Kennedy, 1962.

"I've got a little list, I've got a little list, of society offenders who never would be missed."
Gilbert and Sullivan, *The Mikado*, 1885.

Prior to 1789 the population of France was divided into three estates. The first was the clergy, the second the aristocracy and lastly, the third estate that included everybody else, all but 2% of the population. Royalty were above the system. The Estates General, which had last met in 1614 was convened in June 1789 to try to sort out the national mess resulting from drought, hunger and poverty, and the perilous state of the national economy after

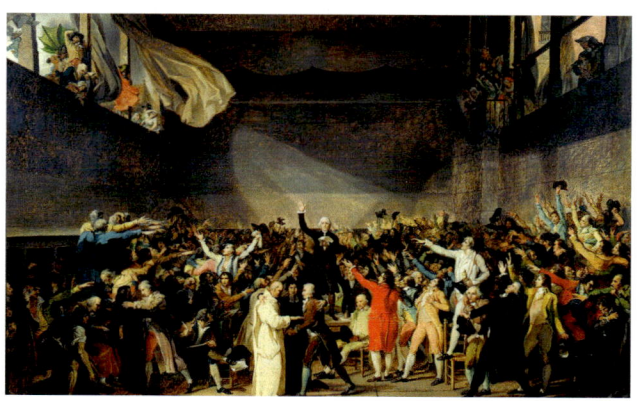

Tennis Court Oath.

3. Nightmare

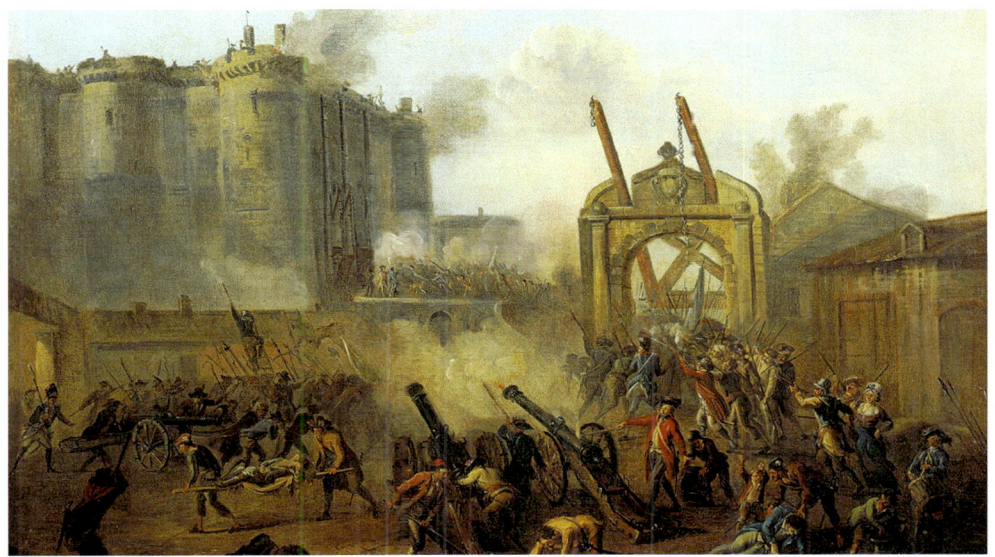

Storming the Bastille.

Louis XVI had overspent in support of the American Revolutionary War, which had ended just six years previously in 1783. Although representing the vast majority of the population, the third estate was inadequately represented and understandably disgruntled. They formed themselves into a National Assembly and when the King tried to stop them by locking and guarding the door to their chamber, they met on 20th June 1789 at an indoor *jeu de paume* court in the city of Versailles near to the palace. An oath was proposed and all but one (a staunch royalist) of the nearly 600 present pledged to remain united and to meet as necessary 'until the constitution of the kingdom is established'. This is remembered as the 'tennis court oath' an important step along the path to revolution. Twenty-four days later on the 14th July 1789 the Bastille prison was stormed and the revolution began.

Massacre

"When one with honeyed words but evil mind persuades the mob, great woes befall the state."

Euripides, Orestes, 408 BC.

The reign of terror and the September massacres

"eleven hundred defenceless prisoners of both sexes and all ages … killed by the populace … four days and nights … darkened by this deed of horror … the air around … tainted by the slain."

Charles Dickens. A Tale of Two Cities, 1859.

When 'the terror' began, is one of those silly things that people argue about. We could copy the attitude of the King in *Alice in Wonderland* and say that "it began when I say it began". Or we could choose between the establishment of the Revolutionary Tribunal in mid-1793 and the September Massacres of 1792. Since the latter is the next point in my story I shall plump for that.

On 19th August 1792 a Prussian army, with the backing of the Emperor of Austria, crossed the border into France with the intention of reversing the revolution. In Paris, uproar and panic immediately ensued with those who supported the revolution and those who opposed it at each other's throats. Danton urged citizens to fight "the traitors within your bosom" and a revolutionary newspaper, the *Orateur du Peuple* declared that "the first war we shall fight will be inside the walls of Paris". One servant of the revolution called out "Once more citizens to arms, to clear the ranks of these vile slaves of tyranny!". It was put about, whether correctly or as what we would now call a conspiracy theory (a conspiracy theory about a conspiracy), that the prisons were stuffed with plotters against the revolution who were waiting for the opportunity to break out and join the anti-revolutionary forces. Those in the prisons to be eliminated included "gilded aristocrats, venal priests, diseased whores, and court lackeys" according to Louis-Sébastien Mercier a writer, dramatist and activist, though said to be 'moderate' (he was himself imprisoned during the terror and opposed the execution of the King, Louis XVI, who nevertheless went to the guillotine on 21st January 1793, exactly 12 dozen years to the month after the English regicide).

The mob of the massacres consisted largely of the so called sans-culottes (the poor men of Paris who couldn't afford the fancy knee breeches favoured by the rich and the aristocrats), along with guardsmen, the fédérés (volunteer guardsmen) and the gendarmes. On the first day of the massacres, which lasted from the 2nd to the 6th of September, Danton, in a speech, declared that "to vanquish them [the enemies of the *patrie*] we need boldness, always boldness, and still more boldness and then France will be saved". He later described the killings as "an indispensable sacrifice". Simon Schama castigates his fellow historians for turning a blind eye to what he refers to as "atrocities unequalled by any others of any party during the French Revolution" and for finding excuses for the slaughter "the scholarly normalization of evil".

The first of the massacres was at the Abbaye prison. A group of priests taken to the prison from the town hall were briefly interrogated and then hacked to pieces, only five of the 19 surviving. The next slaughterhouse was a Carmelite convent where there were 115 victims, and then the Bicêtre where 162 men, youths and boys were slain. At the Salpêtrière the carnage continued, many of the women were raped and some 35 to 40 were murdered, many of them under-aged, including children as young as ten. In all, over the four days, around 1,400 people were butchered, including half of the prisoners in the city (there is considerable variation in the numbers reported). Some blamed Jacques-Louis Marat for encouraging the slaughter and he was dramatically assassinated in his bath by Charlotte Corday as shown in the gruesome painting by Jacques-Louis David. Corday lost her head on the scaffold four days later.

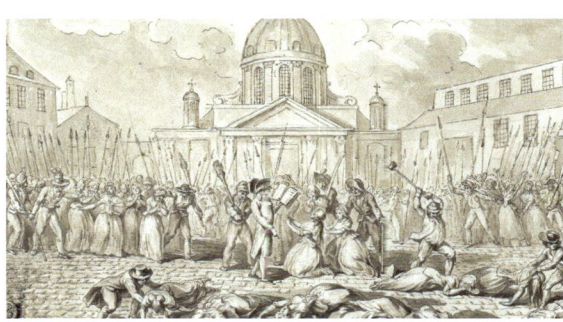

Massacre at the Salpêtriere.

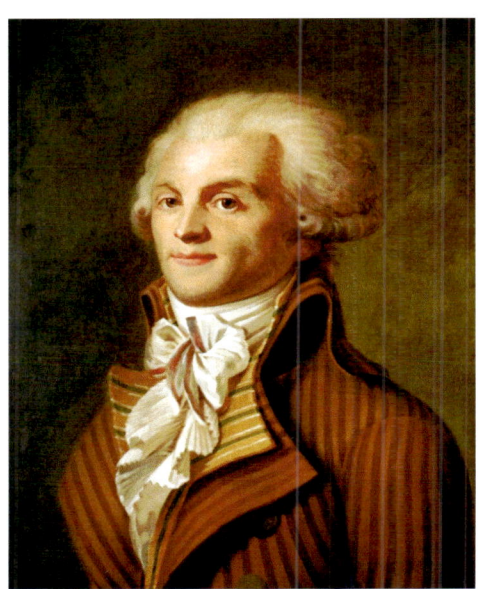

Robespierre.

Robespierre and other theorists of the French Revolution appear to have believed that the elimination of the 'baddies' would leave only the 'goodies' and lead to the perfect world, the 'death to everybody but me and mine'

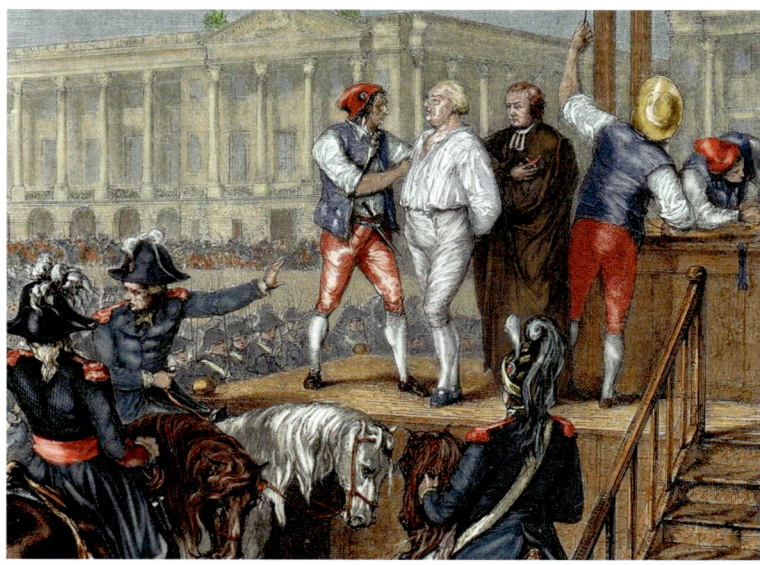

Death of Robespierre.

principle, also subscribed to by 20th century and present day tyrants, although it certainly rebounded on many of them with the inevitable introduction of varying definitions of the words 'me' and 'mine'. Robespierre, as a young judge, had resigned because he couldn't face pronouncing the death sentence. He eventually pronounced that sentence, dispensing with the inconvenience of a trial, on many thousands and, of course, when the tables were turned, he suffered the same fate himself, a victim of his own thanatophoric mania (thanatophoric, from Greek, *thanatos,* death and *phorein*, to bear); you won't find it in a dictionary, it's usually confined to a single terrible disease that ends life almost before it has begun. In all, some 17,000 people fell victim to Dr. Guillotin's 'humanitarian' invention during the revolution. The last use of the guillotine in France was in 1977 and of the rope in England in 1964.

Alors! The Salpêtrière tumbled to a terrible depth,
    like a piece of whalemeat falling to the bottom of the Mariana trench
    to be devoured in that sunless, heatless, hyperbaric void
    by creatures that should not exist
    but do.
AND THEN CAME PINEL.

Chapter 4

A New Dawn

"Begone, you foulest darkness
Hide away you dimming stars
When the day begins
We shall know Success!
Success! Success!"
　　Based on *Nessun Dorma* (final stanza) by Puccini. From the opera *Turandot*.

"We are lucky, even the worst of us, for daylight comes."
　　　　　　　　　　　　Jeanette Winterson. *Lighthousekeeping*, 2006.

Pinel, Esquirol, Duchenne

Philippe Pinel (1745-1826)

The saviour of the Salpêtrière and liberator of the mentally ill. He brought humanity and love to the insane.

"I have deliberately picked the subject which is most obscure and perhaps the most liable to eternal rambling."

　　　　　　　　　　Pinel

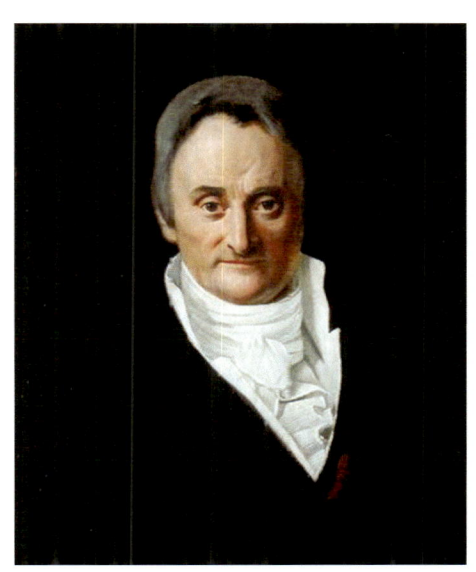

Philippe Pinel.

Philippe Pinel is often spoken of as the world's first psychiatrist. The word psychiatry was first used in Germany at the start of the 19th century but until the end of that century its practitioners were often known as alienists. He was born in Jonquières in what is now the department of Tarn in the south of France. He studied medicine in Toulouse and then in Montpellier but when he moved to Paris in 1778 his qualifications were not recognised, although the Montpellier school had been more prestigious than the Paris one for 600 years (or it would have been had the Paris school existed for that long) but it is true that the Paris faculty had dominated European medicine more recently. So for 15 years he made a living as a writer, translator and editor of the weekly *Health Gazette*. I don't know how he finally wore them down (actually I do, it was the revolution when the initial plan was to abolish medical schools altogether) but they could have enjoyed his exceptional talents for much longer.

The death of a friend from suicide turned him to the study of psychiatry and in 1793 he was appointed physician to the Bicêtre Hospital. The friend had walked out one frosty evening in a fit of madness, clad only in a nightshirt and succumbed to hypothermia, so perhaps it wasn't premeditated suicide, but certainly a malfunction of mindfulness. Pinel was a physician and a professor of medicine before he became a psychiatrist. Ackerknecht, a prominent American medical historian, describes him as the prevailing influence in French medicine of the time. He was not afraid to learn from other cities and other countries; he translated the works of Cullen in Edinburgh and was influenced by the Vienna school. It has been suggested that the appointment to the Bicêtre was not hindered by the fact that he was a strong supporter of the revolution and had influential friends.

There, he was strongly influenced by Jean-Baptiste Pussin and his wife Marguerite who ran the place although they had no qualifications, but they were a pair with great integrity and ability. Pinel later recorded, "I only had the psychiatric patients at the Bicêtre to look after with very restricted facilities … when I moved to the Salpêtrière [in 1795, the same year that the prison side of the Salpêtrière was finally shut down] I was able to resume [his psychiatric career]. Abuses in the service could not possibly have escaped the zeal and sharp eyes of the new supervisor, Mr Pussin. The gothic use of iron chains was abolished." Pussin had followed Pinel to the Salpêtrière and although Pinel is credited with being the first to free the mentally ill from their shackles he acknowledged his indebtedness to Pussin who had done it first at the Bicêtre, though strait jackets were still the order of the day. Pinel went on to

4. A New Dawn

show that when those patients were freed from their iron restraints they rapidly improved and lost their aggressiveness. In the preface to the second edition of his book *Medico-Philosophical Treatise on Mental Alienation* he wrote, "I have very carefully examined the effects which the use of iron chains had on psychiatric patients, compared with the results of their abolition, and I can no longer entertain any doubts about wiser and gentler restraints. The very patients confined to chains for long stretches of years, who had remained in a constant state of rage, thereupon walked about calmly in a simple strait jacket, conversing with everybody, whereas previously nobody could go near them without being in great danger. There was no menacing yelling or shouted threats and their agitated state progressively passed away. They themselves asked for the strait jackets to be put on, and everything came under control." So the patients were insane with frustration having asked, sometimes for years, to be released but never being heeded, an iatrogenic (doctor-made, from Greek *iatros*, a doctor) condition. But which of us has never had that feeling of 'why did it take so long for the penny to drop?' and isn't it so often the things right under our noses that prove the easiest to miss?

So it wasn't a doctor for whom the penny finally dropped. The Pussins are shown attending the patient in the well-known 1876 painting by Tony Robert-Fleury of *Pinel releasing the insane*. This account by Pinel is reminiscent of *Awakenings*, the much praised 1973 book by Oliver Sacks about patients treated with L-DOPA (levodopa) for the parkinsonism (symptoms associated with Parkinson's disease) that followed the pandemic of encephalitis lethargica, which itself was more or less contemporary with the great Spanish influenza pandemic that followed the First World War. Whether the Spanish 'flu was the cause of it all is still debated after 100 years, when I was a medical student in Leeds in the late 1950s and early '60s most of the patients with parkinsonism I saw were said to have post-encephalitic disease.

Pinel's life work became known as 'moral psychiatry', a term I have difficulty with because it uses the word 'moral' in an unusual sense and I am more

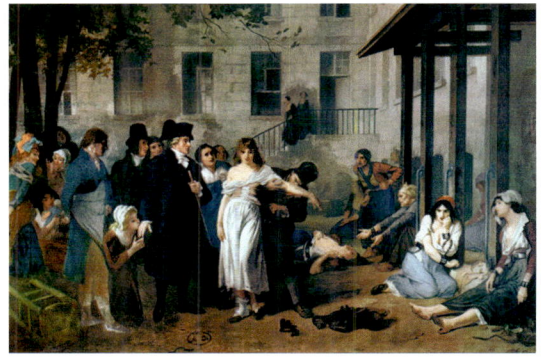

Pinel releasing the insane.

inclined to look to Pinel's compassionate nature. In his writings he eschews fanciful theory and refuses to encroach on religion, basing his principles purely on observation of which he was a dedicated practitioner, visiting his patients often and sometimes more than once a day. His writing is plain to understand, without the complex embroidery of some works. 'Bullshit' was never part of his nature; he would never have found a place in *Private Eye's* 'Pseuds Corner'. It must be remembered that he was working at a time when medicine was only just beginning to emerge from the centuries (almost millennia) long tunnel of obeisance to the doctrines of Hippocrates (around 460-370 BC) and Galen (129-210 AD) and even Pinel seems to feel that he has to discuss the merits of the ancients before moving on. Until 1832 all medical graduates in France ended their graduation thesis with a quote from Hippocrates (there must have been a good trade in suitable Hippocratic quotes). Like Pinel, I have often found psychiatric writings turgid and indecipherable but Pinel's writing has the ring of modernity.

"The educated man has better things to do than sing the praises of his cures."

"The public's concept of medicine is not helped by exaggerated praise any more than by sarcasm."

"It is more important for humanity's sake to find out whether in the present state of the physical sciences one can get any closer to the truth in medicine … by confining oneself over a long period of years to close observation of the course and features of illnesses."

"[The study of Mental Illnesses] calls urgently for the keen attention of genuine observers because of the incoherent and confused hotchpotch it [now] presents."

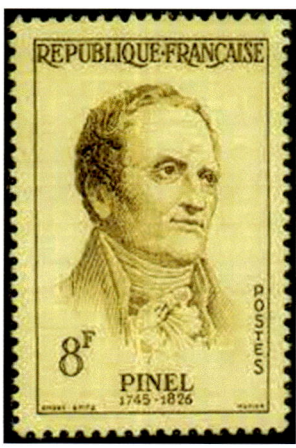

"I cannot avoid giving my most decided sufferage in favour of the moral qualities of maniacs. I have nowhere met, excepting in romances, with fonder husbands, more affectionate parents, more impassioned [people] than in the lunatic asylum, during their intervals of calm and reason."

He talked at length to his patients and tried to understand them, emphasising that when in remission, they were often people of the highest character. Pinel, it could be said, loved the insane. Later, he was criticised for concentrating on the psychological to the exclusion of the biological aspects of his subject but there is no doubt that he fully deserves his high standing in the history of psychiatry, of the Salpêtrière Hospital, of science and of striving humanity.

Pinel received great public acclaim. He was honoured with a postage stamp and appeared on the side of a chocolate box as one of the 'benefactors of humanity', suggesting a considerable degree of 'national treasuredom'. He died in 1826 and, after nearly 200 years, his statue still stands at the entrance to the Salpêtrière. He was, by all accounts, a man of great humanity but I'm not convinced that he has received the recognition he deserves in the 20th and 21st centuries. Before I started looking into the subject of this book I had heard very little about him, and my interest in medical history dates back for many years; I believe that no profession can really know where it is if it doesn't know how it got there. But now he is one of my heroes in the history of my profession and I'm not, by any stretch of the imagination, a psychiatrist.

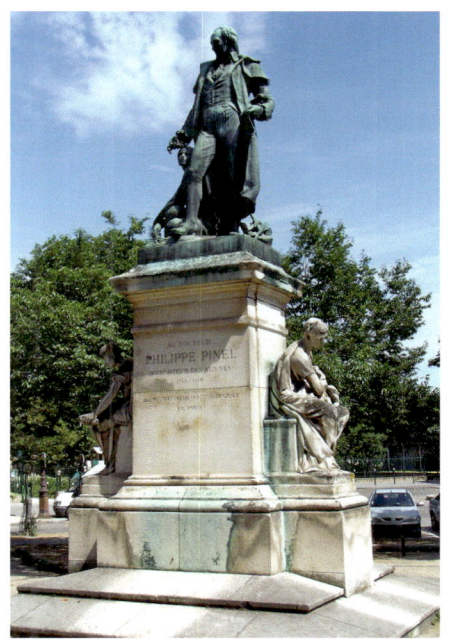

Pinel statue.

Jean-Étienne Dominique Esquirol (1772-1840)

The perpetuation and expansion of Pinel.

"The care of the human mind is the most noble branch of medicine."

Alcysius Sieffert.

I have been unable to locate Aloysius Sieffert (the quotation introduced an article in the *BMJ*) but you would perhaps not be surprised to hear me give a shout for the care of children, who are, after all the single most important item in this world.

Esquirol was a favourite of Pinel and came to outdo him in fame. He was born in Toulouse and attended the medical school in Montpellier before making for

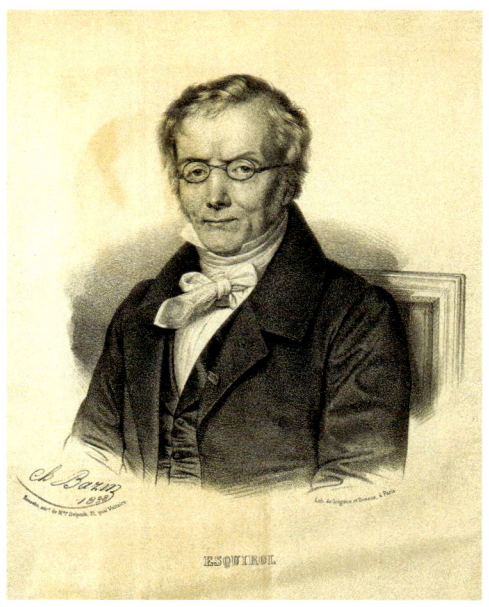

Esquirol.

Paris in 1799. Both Esquirol and Pinel were from the old southern area of Languedoc with its own language of Occitan, and both attended the ancient university of Montpellier, with even now the oldest still active medical school in Europe, founded by Pope Nicholas IV in 1220. So it seems natural that he should head for Pinel and that Pinel should take him on board in what the older man had initially found to be the not exactly welcoming capital. Esquirol arrived in Paris when Pinel had settled into his post at the Salpêtrière. He shared Pinel's bent for psychiatry and Pinel helped him to set up a private asylum which soon developed a very favourable reputation.

He was appointed to the Salpêtrière in 1811 and became an extremely popular teacher, with medical students flocking to his lectures. Between 1810 and 1817, of his own accord, he toured the asylums of France and reported that they were totally inadequate. As an associate of influential politicians he had the ear of government and produced a four point plan to the effect that the mentally ill should be cared for in special hospitals with doctors specifically trained for the job: the advances made in Paris should be spread elsewhere; these hospitals should be of such structural quality that would favour the treatment of their patients and each of them should be run by a doctor who would be firmly in charge. He became Inspector General of Medical Facilities and wrote a textbook of psychiatry *Mental Illnesses considered under the headings Medical, Hygienic and Medico-Legal*, which remained the standard text on psychiatry for half a century. He wrote on the classification of mental illnesses and was instrumental in drafting the 'Law of June 1838' which sought to protect the rights and interests of the mentally ill and is still referred to today. It was said that Esquirol had become more famous throughout France than Pinel whose interest had been confined to the Salpêtrière.

He died in 1840 and his name has been applied to a square, an avenue and a street in Toulouse, Lyon and Paris. There are three Esquirol Hospitals and one Esquirol Clinic. It will be recalled that he attended Théroigne de Méricourt and supplied a diagnosis when she was confined within the Salpêtrière.

Guillaume-Benjamin-Amand Duchenne (1806-1875)

"How is it, one fine morning, Duchenne discovered a disease which probably existed in the time of Hippocrates?"

Jean-Martin Charcot.

"Have you tried to drive a harpoon through a body? Tut, tut my dear sir, you must really pay attention to these details."

Arthur Conan Doyle (1859-1930).

Duchenne is regarded as perhaps the foremost medical scientist of the 19th century. He was often known as Duchenne de Boulogne having been born in that city in 1806 into a long line of seafarers. He introduced the 'de Boulogne' himself to distinguish himself from a member of the Parisian medical elite called Duchesne. His father was a captain in the French navy at a time when that navy was having a spot of bother with a chap called Horatio, and was honoured with the *Légion d'Honneur* by Napoleon. Our Duchenne was born 11 months after Trafalgar, perhaps his father had been in need of time off and a little rest and recuperation, could it be possible that we have to thank Nelson for Duchenne?

Duchenne studied medicine at the University of Paris under such luminaries as Laennec, Magendie, and Dupuytren. Laennec was the person who introduced the stethoscope into medical practice; Magendie was a famous anatomist and physiologist known to all medical students

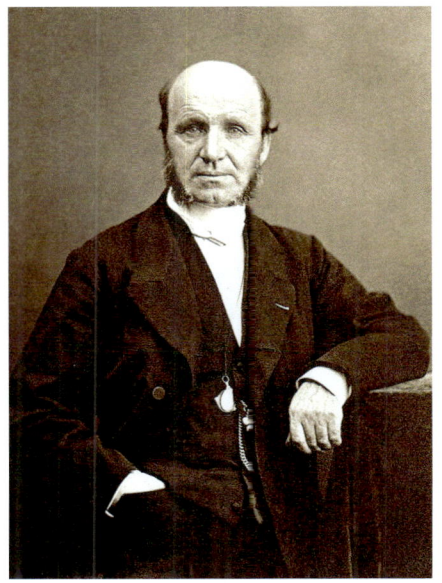

Duchenne.

because of the foramen of Magendie, a structure in the brain, and Dupuytren was a famous surgeon and is remembered for Dupuytren's contracture, a condition of the hand in which hard fibrous nodules develop around the flexor tendons of the fingers. Over a period of years they become thickened and shortened, closing the hand, or more commonly just the little finger. In some it has a hereditary basis and it is said to be more common in people with Scandinavian genes so has been called the Viking disease. My wife had it and so do two of our three children (it seems a strange feature of the language that the accepted term for our children when they are grown up is an oxymoron; adult children. I don't know whether other languages have a suitable word). Many people in Yorkshire are thought to be descendants of the Vikings and Jennifer was highly tickled by the thought she was a Viking. There was DNA evidence to support the contention. Margaret Thatcher had it but in her case, scurrilously or not, it was suggested that the cause was not genes but alcohol. Baron Guillaume Dupuytren (pronounced doo-<u>pwee</u>-tron, not Jupitron as is heard in most English hospitals) was a brilliant surgeon with an enormous practice, chief surgeon at the Hotel-Dieu in Paris and a talented teacher. He gained much kudos from treating Napoleon's piles, the pain from which was reported to have influenced the Battle of Waterloo. Napoleon made him a baron.

On qualifying in 1831, Duchenne returned home to Boulogne and spent ten years in general practice. Soon after his return he married a young Boulogne woman, but she died of puerperal sepsis (infection of the womb) soon after giving birth to his only son. In her grief and her anger his mother-in-law blamed him and widely publicised that fact around Boulogne, she took over the care of the infant and Duchenne didn't see his son again for over 30 years. He married again in 1839 to a woman whose outgoing personality is said to have been the opposite of his own introspective nature. He returned to Paris in 1842 after his practice and his marriage had deteriorated. But he wasn't welcomed back to Paris. Some apparently found him a little odd and some of the elite of Parisian medicine looked down on him as an unsophisticated provincial with a Boulogne accent. He never got a job in any of the Paris hospitals, perhaps because he knew the score and didn't bother applying for one, so in order to make a living he went back into general practice, but that wasn't a conspicuous success either, because he didn't seem to spend much time in the practice. Instead he would be a regular visitor at the Paris hospitals, particularly the Salpêtrière, examining patients, making copious notes and if necessary following them from hospital to hospital.

4. A New Dawn

Duchenne was finally taken on by some prominent physicians and surgeons, including Armand Trousseau, a prominent physician at the Salpêtrière and Paul Broca (see later). On exactly what terms he was taken on is not clear but it allowed him access to the patients. He also began a close friendship with Charcot. He initiated and developed the use of electricity in medical diagnosis and treatment. He invented what became known as Duchenne's electrical apparatus and with it he was able to show that some babies had suffered, during birth, damage to the brachial plexus, the collection of nerves high up inside the armpit as they leave the spinal cord to supply the muscles of the arm, usually damaged, if damaged at all, in a difficult delivery. He introduced the term 'brachial plexus palsy'. Some years later Wilhelm Heinrich Erb (1840-1921), who worked at the Universities of Leipzig and Heidelberg, added to the subject and it became known as Erb's palsy or Erb-Duchenne palsy.

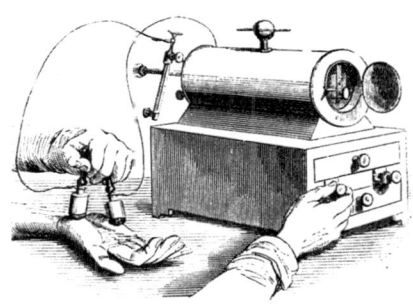

Duchenne's electrical apparatus.

Duchenne is now recognised as the founder of clinical electrophysiology. He was also one of the founders of clinical photography. Photography itself had begun in France with Joseph Nicéphore Niépce and Louis Daguerre working together. The French medical microscopist Alfred François Donné had used it soon after Daguerre had presented his findings to the Académie des Sciences in 1839 and the first clinical photograph of a patient (with a large goitre or swelling of the thyroid gland in the neck) was in the mid-1840s in Scotland. Duchenne produced a set of clinical photographs in 1862 when he published a book *Le Mécanisme de la Physionomie Humaine* (The Mechanism of Human Facial Expression). He would apply an electric current to various parts of the face, causing considerable discomfort and photograph the resulting facial expressions, locating the responsible muscles. That may or may not have been of great value to the human race but it interested Charles Darwin (1809-82) who published his *The Expression of the Emotions in Man and Animals* in 1872. Darwin wrote to Duchenne to ask how much he would charge to give permission to publish some of his pictures and Duchenne wrote back to say that between men of science there could be no charge.

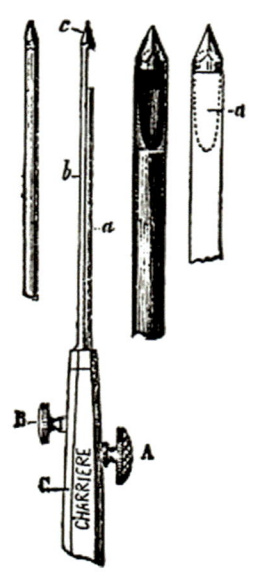

Muscle biopsy needle.

Duchenne is best known, of course, for the muscle disease that affects boys, carries his name and was the object of the rhetorical inquiry by Charcot with which this chapter began. He invented a muscle biopsy needle. With no local anaesthetic his contemporaries questioned the ethics of the procedure and indeed Duchenne seems to have been a driven researcher with sparse regard for the difficulties for himself or his patients. The new device was called, sarcastically, 'Duchenne's histological harpoon', harpoon obviously harks back in a cynical way to his seafaring origins and points to the apparently brutal manner of its use. The physicians of Paris had not taken him to their hearts but he continued with his research and was able to show that the increase in bulk of the muscles of the calves characteristic of this disease is due, not to an increase in muscle cells but to an increase of fat within the muscles indicating degeneration of the muscle tissue. He called it 'pseudohypertrophic muscular dystrophy' a name that has stood the test of time, though today it is usually known as Duchenne type muscular dystrophy or DMD. It affects only boys because it is inherited in an X-linked (or sex-linked) manner (see addendum for non-medical readers).

Duchenne died in 1875 at the age of 69. He had achieved international recognition and was invited into the courts of the Queen Empress of the British Empire (Queen Victoria) and of the King of Spain. Towards the end of his life he blossomed socially, often inviting for dinner some of the cream of Parisian medical society including in particular Charcot and Alfred Vulpian (1826-87), the latter being the discoverer of adrenaline and first to use the term atrial fibrillation (see later). He died after a stroke in August 1875 but he didn't die alone.

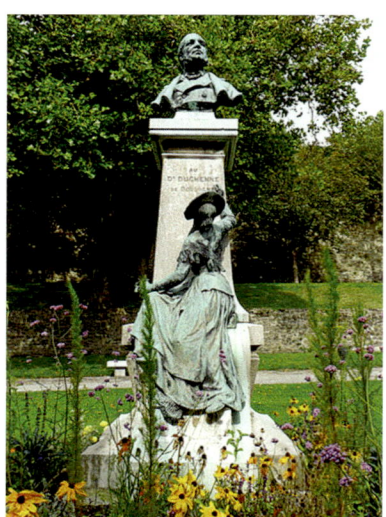

Duchenne's memorial.

4. A New Dawn

Charcot and Professor Charles Potain, a mutual friend and prominent cardiologist, never left him alone in his final days, taking it in turns to stay with him. There is a bust on an angelic column in a public garden in Boulogne and the Duchenne Hospital dominates the main hospital complex in the city.

Charles Dickens (1812-70) was a close contemporary of Duchenne and a confirmed Francophile. He was particularly fond of Boulogne, sang its praises and lived there for several years. There is a *Rue Charles Dickens* in Boulogne. Whether he and Duchenne ever met, I don't know.

Addendum for non-medical readers

X-linked inheritance

Women have two X chromosomes, one from each parent and men have one X and one Y (smaller) chromosome, the X from their mother and the Y from their father. The DMD gene is carried on an X chromosome. The mother of a child with DMD has one normal X chromosome and one abnormal (carrying the DMD gene). Embryos with two abnormal Xs do not survive early pregnancy. Because the inheritance is X-linked, *recessive* a normal X, will always 'trump' an abnormal one so women can only be carriers of the disease but they will give their abnormal X to half of their sons. Since the son receiving that X chromosome has no other X to 'trump' it he will have the disease. Other diseases or conditions with X-linked recessive inheritance include haemophilia, red-green colour blindness and several rare neurological diseases. Queen Victoria was a carrier for haemophilia. A worldwide study published in 2020 showed a prevalence rate of DMD within the community at all ages of 5 per 100,000 males and an incidence (rate in newborn boys) of 21 per 100,000. The cause is a change (mutation) in the dystrophin gene causing dystrophin not to be produced or produced in an inactive form. Dystrophin is a protein essential to maintain the health of muscle fibres. Modern care has improved lengths of survival and, as with all single gene diseases, there is hope of eventual gene therapy.

Chapter 5

Daybreak

Jean-Martin Charcot (1825-1893)
King of the Salpêtrière and Founder of Modern Neurology

"A great person attracts great people and knows how to hold them together."
					Johan Wolfgang von Goethe (1749-1832).

In 2011 a monograph outlined the biographies of twelve of Charcot's distinguished interns, none of whom I am ashamed to say are known to me, I shall tell you about the Charcot acolytes I do know about. I only mention the monograph to illustrate the number of distinguished doctors trained by Charcot.

Charcot was the towering figure in French medicine and to a large extent in European medicine, of the 19th century and is recognised as the founder of modern neurology. He was born in Paris in 1825, his life overlapped with that of Pinel by a year. His parents were Simon-Pierre Charcot and his wife Jeanne-Georgette, his father was a carriage builder and Charcot's parents were living with his mother's parents when Charcot was born. He was one of four brothers, one of whom remained in the family business whilst the two

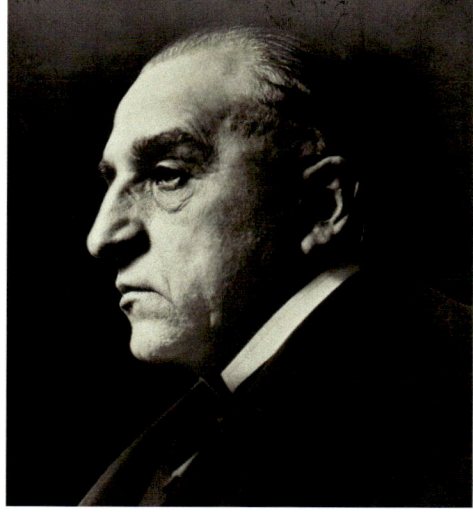

Charcot.

5. Daybreak

others achieved high rank in the army, one being killed in battle. It is said that when they were children his father promised to fund for university the son who did best at school and Jean-Martin was that one.

In childhood and throughout life Charcot, it seems, was a quiet, reserved and self-sufficient character. He had a talent for drawing and caricature and would illustrate his lectures with his own medical artwork. Some years after he died a former pupil produced a book *Charcot, the artist*. Although he was reserved with people he loved animals and bristled at any whiff of animal cruelty; he even had a pet monkey. He was not religious but tolerant of the faiths of others. In medicine he believed in the well trained physician "A physician is only as good a clinician as he is a pathologist". He would not take instructions except from his wife and then only on such occasions as when he was told it was time to stop working and retire to bed.

Charcot spent his early days as a student in the Bohemian atmosphere of the Paris Latin Quarter. At that time medicine was regarded as a profession for the sons of the middle class and there were many of them, about two and a half thousand medical students at the Paris school, with consequently much competition and jostling for a place. Much was left to the students' assertiveness to seek out good clinical teachers and the less assertive could possibly qualify having barely set eyes on a patient. Only the better students became externs and even fewer interns at a hospital. Obtaining a medical degree could be a long and gruelling process, in the late 1880s fewer than 10% got their degree in less than five years and well over that proportion were still plugging away after eleven years or more (reminiscent of the very popular old film *Doctor in the House* in which Kenneth More's character Richard Grimsdyke is so fond of being a medical student that he deliberately fails his exams so that he can carry on almost indefinitely). Once qualified, progression up the ladder for those who wished to pursue a hospital career was difficult, highly competitive and often painful. The final steps in the progression were often not achieved until nearing forty. Charcot was a good, even very good student, but not outstanding and he had some reverses at examinations, which may have been the fault of the examination system rather than the result of his own inadequacies.

Charcot progressed through the hospital ranks of extern and intern and came under the tutelage of Professor P.F.O. Rayner who was a man of considerable fame and influence, having treated the Emperor Napoleon III and become Dean of the Faculty of Medicine at the University of Paris. He supported Charcot at the *Agrégation* exams when, it seems, not only your knowledge and competence but your professorial supporters were important. Charcot passed in 1860 having failed two years earlier (see the examination controversy of 1872 in the chapter on Babinski). Charcot had his own views about these exams which he thought were unfair. He was in favour of strict but fair exams up to the point of qualification but against such competitive exams for postgraduates which some candidates would be taking quite late in life. He thought that such matters should be assessed on the basis of past performance.

Charcot was appointed chief physician at the Salpêtrière in 1862. It is not unusual to look upon the history of the Salpêtrière as that before and after 1862. One of the first things Charcot did after he arrived there was to set up a pathology laboratory. His research, in the main, consisted of correlating clinical with pathological findings. He was appointed Professor of Pathological Anatomy in 1870. One of the things that most excited him about the post at the Salpêtrière was the vast number of patients he could study, many of them with chronic neurological disease. He looked upon it as a vast museum of living pathology from which he could learn so much.

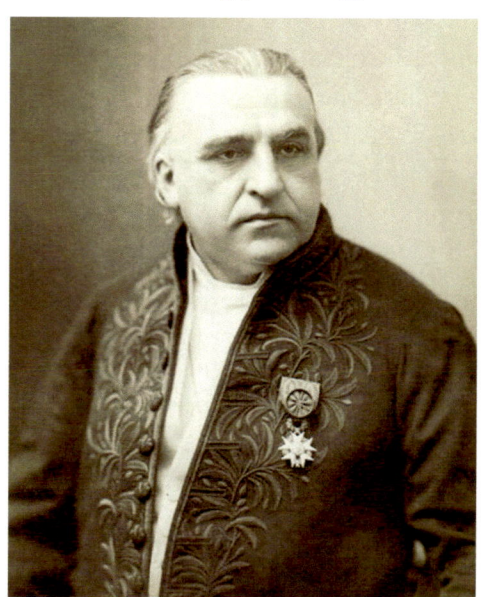

Charcot.

Charcot rarely did ward rounds. There is a sketch by an unknown artist of Charcot doing a ward round and showing Bourneville waving a thermometer. Bourneville was one of the first to use a clinical thermometer (see later). Charcot would sit in his office and have the patients brought to him, the interns would present the patients one by one and go through the clinical findings. He would ask the patient to move or speak but otherwise would remain silent. This would be repeated with a succession of patients. His thoughts, presumably, were not considered relevant to or for the patient. Today, of course, when

5. Daybreak

patient-doctor interaction is all-important it would not be tolerated. Some writers, however, report instances of Charcot's caring and kindness to patients. Charcot certainly seemed to have a Napoleon complex as is easily seen in some of his photographs. After the session, Charcot would get into his carriage and be driven home, still not having spoken, apart from a few instructions to the interns. Despite all this his interns, or the ones who left a record of it, were fiercely loyal to him as he was to them. Many of them would themselves become prominent within the profession.

Charcot became known internationally as a great teacher. Ambitious young doctors from far and wide would come to Paris to sit at the feet of the great Charcot. He would go to great pains to get his points across and would illustrate his lectures with his own graphical skills on the blackboard. He was among the first to use a projector, he never read from a script and he would prepare his lectures with great care and commit to memory what he was going to say and his juniors would record what he said and prepare it for publication. He was not an eloquent speaker being surprisingly withdrawn in that respect but according to Gilles de la Tourette he, "never learned how to speak without saying anything". He would lecture on Friday mornings and give clinical presentations on Tuesday mornings. In his Tuesday presentations he would assess the patient and come to a diagnosis in front of the students not having seen the patient before. In his lectures he would, if necessary, himself adopt the postures needed to illustrate the various neurological disorders. His lectures would also be attended by writers, artists and other celebrities of the city and across Europe. Sigmund Freud spent four months learning from Charcot and was greatly impressed by him (see later). As his reputation grew he would have audiences of several hundreds. He was a talented linguist and could draw upon his vast knowledge of medical reports in English, German and Italian as well as his native French.

One of the best known paintings in medical history is *A clinical lesson at the Salpêtrière* painted in 1887 by André Brouillet, an academic artist who specialised in genre paintings (scenes from ordinary life), portraits, landscapes and oriental art. It shows his long-time patient Blanche Wittman being induced by Charcot to have an 'hysterical fit'. Babinski (see below) is standing behind the patient ready to catch her and onlookers include Gilles de la Tourette, Pierre Marie, Édouard Brissaud, Désiré-Magloire Bourneville and Charcot's son, Jean-Baptiste, each of whom will feature later. It is currently to be found

Salpêtrière

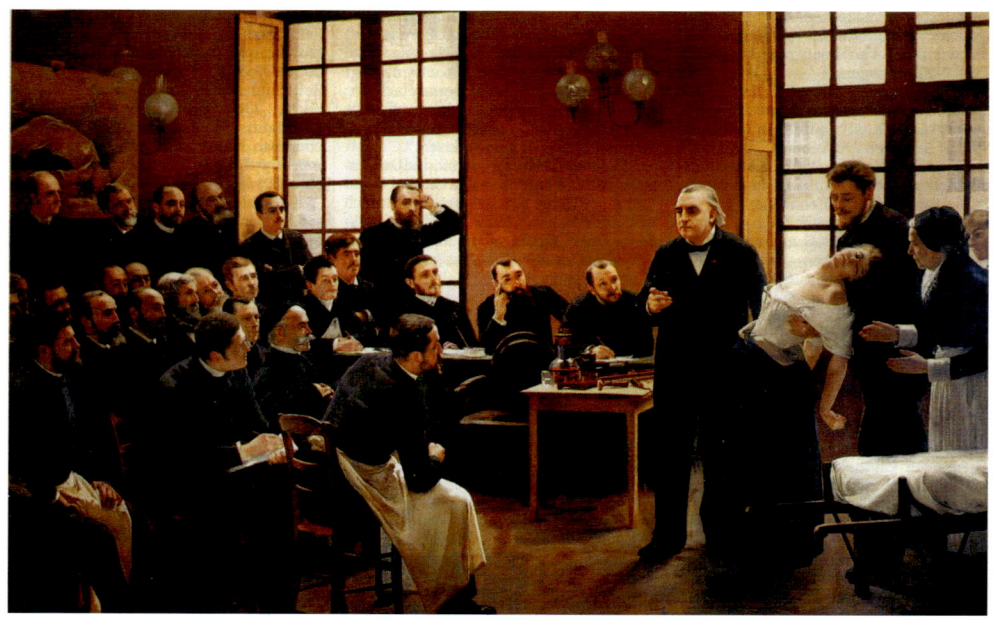

A clinical lesson at the Salpêtrière.

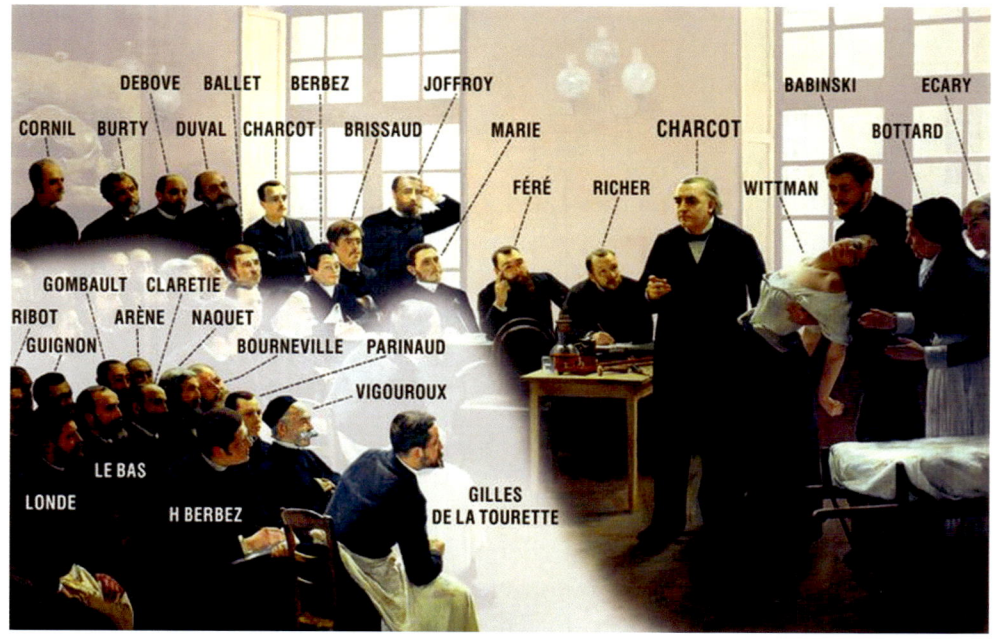

hanging in a corridor of the Descartes University in Paris outside the entrance to the Museum of the History of Medicine but it, apparently, was only returned to Paris after spending some years unnoticed in corners of Nice and Lyon. Today the painting would not receive ethical approval (where was the 'me too' movement in 1887?). A young woman in a sexually provocative pose being scrutinised eagerly by a group of male doctors having been induced into having a fit by their ringleader? Not in the 21st century.

Marguerite Bottard (1822-1906)

"Virtue is bold and goodness never fearful."

Shakespeare, *Measure for Measure*.

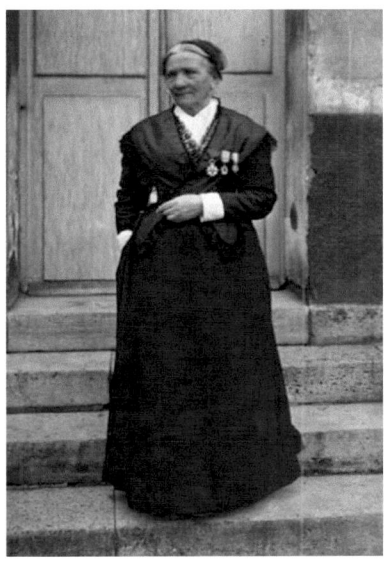

Marguerite Bottard.

Also in the picture, caring for the patient, is Charcot's chief nurse Marguerite Bottard. She predated Charcot at the Salpêtrière by 21 years, knew him as an intern and as *Chef de Service* and throughout his professorship, and was chief nurse at the time he died. She was born in 1822 into an impoverished peasant family in Burgundy the fourth of 15 children. She came to the Salpêtrière in 1841 at the age of 19 as a ward cleaner, general dogsbody and all round factotum. At that time nursing duties were carried out, or not carried out, by nuns who at times it was said, would pay more attention to their religious observances than to the patients. Marguerite slid into the role of assistant care giver, by 1852 she was assistant chief nurse on a psychiatric section where she became known for her kindness and efficiency and by 1861 was chief nurse. Charcot took over the ward in 1870 and she worked with him until he died in 1893. She made the Salpêtrière her whole life never leaving it except to accompany patients but in doing the latter she ran into grave danger in Paris in the Franco-Prussian war of 1870. She looked after the needs of the interns and became loved by everyone. Gilles de la Tourette called her Mum Bottard and she became the mother of the department to whom they would all run when in trouble or in need of a shoulder to cry on, including the boss, Charcot. She never married and had no children of her own but she cared for a nephew. The man she seems to have loved died in a cholera epidemic in 1849.

Marguerite was much honoured, receiving the Montyon Prize (for virtue) and becoming a *Chevalier d'Honneur*. Much later Charcot's daughter wrote of an incident when Charcot was entertained for dinner in the doctors' mess. The dinner went on late and became quite noisy, the professor being not the least of the noise makers. When he said good morning to the sister the following day she smiled sweetly and said "The interns made such a noise last night we were unable to sleep" knowing full well who was the main culprit (so he wasn't entirely strait-laced). Marguerite celebrated 50 years of service in 1891 when Charcot made an eye-wetting speech of praise and Gilles de la Tourette wrote a letter to a newspaper in similar vein. After Charcot died in 1893 she worked first with Édouard Brissaud the temporary professor and then with Fulgence Raymond, Charcot's successor. On retiring after 60 years of service in 1901 she lived in the *Pavillon des Reposantes* (for the resting) in the grounds of the hospital, a facility originally provided by Cardinal Mazarin. She died in 1906 aged 84.

Charcot and non-neurological diseases

"The true genius is a mind of large general powers accidentally determined to some particular direction."

Dr Samuel Johnson, 1780.

Charcot wasn't confined to neurology before he became the world's first professor of neurology in 1882, although his position as first professor of neurology has been disputed; apparently Charles Karmer Mills was clinical Professor of Nervous Diseases at the medical school of the University of Pennsylvania (the first American university, founded by Benjamin Franklin), in 1872. Charcot wrote his MD thesis in 1853 on 'asthenic gout'. Before that time all chronic joint disease was regarded as gout. Charcot distinguished between gout and what we now call rheumatoid arthritis. The term rheumatoid arthritis was introduced by Alfred Baring Garrod (1819-1907) a physician at University College Hospital, London and later King's College Hospital, it had previously been known as rheumatic gout. Charcot later performed further studies on gout (as now defined) confirming, after Garrod, the importance of uric acid as both a cause and a test for the disease. Charcot's joint, or neuropathic arthropathy, is a degenerative joint disease due to repeated injury to a weight bearing joint after loss of feeling in the joint. Charcot described it in tabes dorsalis (syphilis of the spine) but it is seen today in diabetes and other causes of sensory loss. Many rheumatologists now accept Charcot as one of the founders of their discipline. There are many Charcot eponyms, most of them not in current use, the second edition of Stedman's *Medical Eponyms* lists 23. The better known ones, to me, are: Charcot's joint; Charcot's triad (right upper abdominal pain, fever and jaundice in acute infection of the biliary tract secondary to gallstones); Charcot's neurological triad (nystagmus – rhythmical rapid, involuntary eye movements; tremor and scanning speech in multiple sclerosis) and Charcot-Marie-Tooth disease (see later). Motor neurone disease was at one time known as Charcot's disease. He also wrote a book about the diseases of old age and was the first to describe intermittent claudication (pain in the leg on walking due to narrowing of the main artery to the leg). He and Bouchard described cerebral aneurysms as a cause of intracranial bleeding.

Charcot's neurology

Charcot addressed one of his packed audiences as follows: *"… the number… here today is proof… of my belief… that this vast emporium of human suffering… might become a seat of theoretical and clinical instruction, of uncontested utility."*

J-M Charcot, Lectures on the diseases of the nervous system, delivered at La Salpêtrière. Volume 1 (preliminary observations), MDCCCLXXVII (1878). Translated by George Sigerson.

Parkinson's disease

Charcot's method of pursuing research was the anatomo-clinical method that he expanded after Laennec. He would have, for each patient, carefully preserved clinical details and would correlate them with autopsy findings including histology, something Laennec did not have. He also made extensive use of photography, a habit he acquired from Duchenne.

Charcot was the first to distinguish reliably between what we now call Parkinson's disease and other neurological conditions, in particular multiple sclerosis. He was always a stickler for giving credit where it was due and insisted that what James Parkinson in 1817 had called *paralysis agitans* should now be called Parkinson's disease. James Parkinson (1755-1824) was himself a man whose worthiness appears to merit more than his confinement, or definition, by a single disease. Born in Shoreditch, London, the son of an apothecary and surgeon, he qualified in medicine at The London Hospital after being apprenticed to his father. He practiced locally and was one of the first to operate for appendicitis, with his son John. He also designed a truss for hernias. He wrote his famous account of 'the shaking palsy' in 1817. In addition to his medical career he campaigned for social reform, in particular for extension of the suffrage, for the rights of the poor and the mentally ill, and for protections for child workers. He was also one of the first fossil collectors. He advanced the science of palaeontology and was a founder member of the British Geological Society (I've just come across a word new to me, oryctologist, it seems to be used as a name for fossil collectors or those who give names to fossils. But it's not in any of my dictionaries and if you try to look it up on Google you get a definition of proctology). Amusingly, he wrote under the name of 'Old Hubert'.

Multiple sclerosis

In 1866 and 1868 Charcot and Vulpian elucidated the clinical and pathological aspects of multiple sclerosis. Charcot introduced the name, multiple sclerosis (*sclerose en plaques*) and was able to distinguish clearly for the first time between this disease and paralysis agitans. Charcot and Vulpian examined the sclerotic plaques in the brain and correlated the pathological findings with the clinical features of the disease.

Motor neurone disease

In 1865 Charcot examined a woman at the Salpêtrière and thought he'd found a new disease. He hoped he would be able to define this disease as well as Duchenne had previously defined tabes dorsalis. On clinical and pathological grounds he called the new disease amyotrophic lateral sclerosis. That name remains in use today but it is more often called motor neurone disease (MND). In America it may be called Lou Gehrig's disease after a big hitter with the New York Yankees baseball team who developed the disease. It is a disease of the motor neurones of the brain and spinal cord (see the addendum to the Chapter on Babinski). Over 330,000 people worldwide have

MND. It is more common in men. The lifetime risk is around 1 in 350 for men and 1 in 470 for women. It is probably the disease most doctors would name as their most feared.

Charcot-Marie-Tooth disease
See under Pierre Marie.

Hysteria
"The use of the word, hysteria, is deplorable."
        Georges Guillain. In *J M Charcot, His Life His Work*. 1959.

The word, hysteria, comes from the Greek for a womb or uterus (*hustera*). In ancient Egypt the uterus was bizarrely imagined to be not fixed in the body but capable of moving around and this wandering uterus was considered to be the cause of hysteria which consequently was thought to affect only women. During the middle ages the peripatetic uterus hypothesis was abandoned and instead it was attributed to sin and demonic possession, and exorcism seemed the logical treatment. Towards the end of the 18th century Thomas Sydenham, a physician from Dorset who became known as the English Hippocrates, declared that hysteria was a matter of the emotions. Charcot, and later Freud, devoted much time to the subject. During the 20th century medical minds turned away from hysteria and to diagnosing conversion symptoms, depression, or anxiety and in 1980 hysteria was declared a non-diagnosis when the word was removed from the medical vocabulary. It was dropped from the all-important *Diagnostic and Statistical Manual* (DSM) of Mental Disorders of the American Psychiatric Association which lists all approved psychiatric diagnoses.

At the Salpêtrière people with epilepsy and those with a diagnosis of hysteria were treated together and Charcot was put in charge of that section so he had a lot of patients with those diagnoses. It also gave the 'hysterics', who were susceptible to suggestion, the opportunity to copy the patients with epilepsy. Charcot lectured a lot about hysteria. Later his ideas were criticised but he seems to have been aware of and to have confronted the main criticisms. His most fervent critics were in the medical school in Nancy in northeast France where his use of hypnotism to treat hysteria was vociferously opposed. Babinski (see later) emphasised the importance of suggestion in hysteria and introduced the word pithiatism from the Greek words for suggestion and cure. That word soon became defunct.

Charcot had several well-known 'hysterics' as long term residents at the hospital and it was often claimed that he trained them to perform for him, which he denied. The best known was the one in the famous painting, Marie (Blanche) Wittman. She was born in Paris in 1859, the daughter of a Swiss carpenter who treated her badly and who was admitted to an asylum as insane and a linen maid mother. In early childhood she developed presumably elective (or selective) mutism and she stopped speaking which lasted for five years. Perhaps poor Blanche's situation made her perpetually very anxious or perhaps she'd discovered that speaking to people was not a rewarding thing to do and she was better off keeping her mouth shut. She was said to be subject to 'fits of anger', almost certainly breath holding, all in all the picture of a very frustrated little girl. When Blanche had one of her fits of anger her mother would throw cold water at her, that might sound like child abuse but it was probably a recognised treatment at the time. The pre-eminent English speaking physician of the Victorian-Edwardian era Sir William Osler, advocated a treatment for frequent breath holding that he'd been given as a tip by Dr. Sydney Ringer at University College London (yes, the great Osler acted on tips). Ringer was known for Ringer's solution, a mixture of salts for intravenous infusion. His tip was to treat frequent breath holding by giving the child a warm bath three times a day during which the child's chest and back would be sponged with cold water. During an attack though, the water was best "dashed into the child's face". It seems unlikely that Blanche's mother would have been able to run a hot bath in the slums of Paris in the 19th century. She probably knew about breath holding though before Osler did, even though she didn't speak his language; she obviously knew about water throwing. He called it 'spasmodic laryngitis' but in his textbook *The Principles and Practice of Medicine* first published in 1893 and the 'medical bible' for doctors and medical students for over 50 years, he wrote "mothers call it holding the breath"(sometimes the profession catches up with the public). Blanche was admitted to the Salpêtrière under Charcot's care at the age of 18. She became known as 'The queen of the hysterics'. A study of the available evidence by doctors in Madrid in 2016 concluded that her attacks were 'psychogenic non-epileptic seizures', really Charcot's own diagnosis put in more up-to-date language, the type of language that makes people believe, falsely, that they're one ahead of their predecessors. In 2006 a novel *The Story of Blanche and Marie* by Per Olav Enquist told of Blanche being taken on by Marie Curie as a laboratory assistant after Charcot died and losing an arm and two legs from the effects of radiation. The propriety of the relationships between Blanche and both Charcot and Curie was also called into question. The story was praised as a novel but attracted considerable scepticism as history. In 2007 in a letter to the medical journal *The Lancet,* Enquist was accused of slandering (libelling surely?) Blanche and two icons of science, Charcot and Curie. Blanche died in 1913. Curie herself died of aplastic anaemia (bone marrow failure) due to radiation exposure.

Another of Charcot's patients who became famous was Jane Avril. Born Jeanne Louise Beadon in 1868, the daughter of a prostitute and an Italian aristocrat, she had a troubled childhood and was admitted to the Salpêtrière in 1882 with multiple tics and 'hysterical fits'. She later achieved fame as a dancer, first at the *Moulin Rouge* and then at the *Jardin de Paris* on the Champs-Elysées. She would introduce tic-like movements into her dancing, whether involuntarily or not seems uncertain, and she would dance the can-can. She was the subject of a well-known painting by Toulouse-Lautrec and was portrayed on film by Zsa Zsa Gabor in 1952 and by Nicole Kidman in 2001. She died in poverty in 1943.

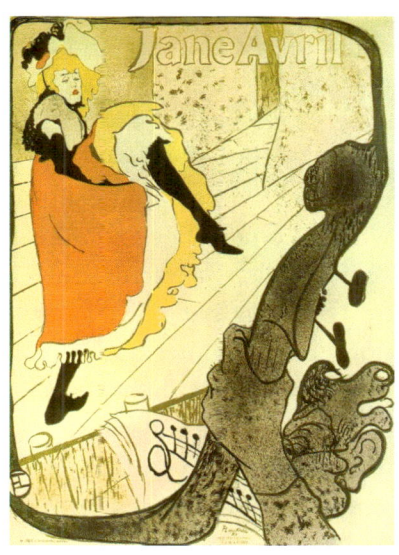

Poster by Toulouse-Lautrec.

Like many of his contemporaries, Charcot often showed a healthy disdain for the 'cures' of the day. Effective therapeutics has been, by and large, a phenomenon born of the 20th century and advances in chemistry. In 1901, Osler listed the medicines he thought effective, there were six: quinine, iron, mercury, iodide of potassium, opium and digitalis. Charcot was willing to give new remedies a try but not in the sense of a modern therapeutic trial. For Parkinson's disease he prescribed rest, hyoscine and camphor, and he used colchicine for gout and mercury-containing compounds for syphilis. His therapeutic repertoire also included silver nitrate, iron, herbane and zinc oxide. For physical therapies he used hydrotherapy, electrotherapy, muscle strengthening exercises and suspension therapy (hanging patients up in a brace to straighten the spine). The latter was intended to relieve pressure on and stretch the spine. Its use on Alphonse Daudet, a celebrated writer and friend of the Charcot family, caused a rift with the patient. Charcot later stopped using it. He also used various forms of minor psychotherapy.

In 1864 Charcot married a rich widow, Augustine Victoire Durvis, the daughter of the owner of a fashionable clothing house, *Maison Laurent Richard*, later tailors to the royal court (I've been unable to discover whether Yves Saint Laurent was related). As his fame grew and he attracted private patients in Paris and from around the world, Charcot became rich of his own right. They rented, and then bought, a house in Neuilly sur Seine, a fashionable and well-heeled suburb to the west of Paris, at that time regarded as 'country', and spent their summers there. In Paris at his regular Tuesday soirees with his wife he entertained an Emperor (of Brazil), Russian grand dukes, a cardinal, politicians, artists, writers, and high ranking police together with his colleagues and pupils such as Marie, Babinski, Gilles de la Tourette, Bourneville, Brissaud and others. He knew Louis Pasteur (1822-95), their professional lives did not cross very much but Pasteur would visit Charcot's home and on one occasion at the Academy of Medicine, when Pasteur's anti-rabies vaccine had been under attack, he strongly defended Pasteur repeating that the vaccine was a thing of great beauty both as a scientific and as a moral entity. Even today the 'antivaxers', those who would throw away probably the single advance in medicine that has saved more lives than any other, are still with us over 230 years later (Pinel began a smallpox vaccination clinic in Paris in the 1790s).

In June 1893 Charcot became involved in 'The Panama Scandal' which involved the financial affairs and bankruptcy of the Panama Canal Company in Paris. Ministers and members of parliament were accused of bribery and corruption and millions of Francs were lost by thousands of people. One of the prominent accused was one Dr Cornelius Hertz, a French American physician, entrepreneur and businessman. He was in England in June 1893 and was called to Paris for trial but claimed to be unfit to travel and Charcot was part of a team of doctors sent to examine him. Much to the disgust of the press and the public they found Hertz not fit to travel, causing a great outcry. The stress on Charcot had been noticeable and in August his wife recruited several of his young friends

5. Daybreak

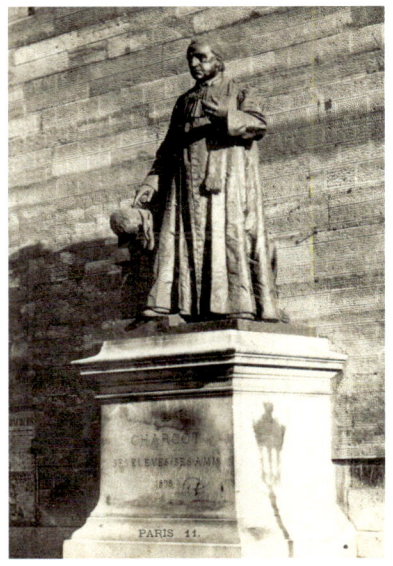

Charcot statue.

to accompany him on a trip to the Morvan lake region of Burgundy. They stayed at a rural inn where his companions were called by the innkeeper's wife at 3.00am to find him sweaty and breathless. The two young physicians among them diagnosed pulmonary oedema due to coronary thrombosis with left heart failure and he died within a few hours. His coffin was placed in the St. Louis Chapel at the Salpêtrière for patients to pay their respects alongside the family, medical and nursing staff, as well as scientific, political, artistic and other dignitaries from France and elsewhere. A statue was put at the entrance to the hospital but during the Second World War it was melted down by the Vichy government in aid of the nazi war effort. Charcot is recognised as the founder of modern neurology, many would include Duchenne as co-founder and Charcot would refer to Duchenne as *'mon maître en neurologie'* which I choose to translate as, 'the one who taught me neurology'.

Charcot's genius, as with so many geniuses, lay in seeing what others did not see. Before Charcot the Salpêtrière was an unattractive place for students and young doctors. It was some distance from the medical school and many students simply couldn't be bothered to get there. For young doctors it was full of 'incurables' and working there didn't much advance the c.v. Where others saw a wastebin of discarded humanity, Charcot saw a vast 'museum of living pathology' to be sorted out and made sense of. He rummaged through the 'dustbin' and found diamonds and from the diamonds he created a beautiful tiara. He entered a run-down peripheral theatre and left a West End full of stars (note that I've said nothing about compassion as a motive, how much it was a motive I'm simply not sure).

The Biological Society of Paris

La Société de Biologie de Paris was founded in 1848 and Charcot was a member from 1851. It was a multidisciplinary society with members from a variety of related professions: anatomy, physiology, anthropology, medicine, surgery and chemistry. It was a place for meeting, sharing views and intellectual stimulation, based on the College de France and the Paris Medical School and there was cross fertilisation of ideas between clinicians, laboratory based scientists and those concerned with public health matters.

Edmé Félix Alfred Vulpian (1826-1887)

"And my heart beats so that I can hardly speak."

Irving Berlin, 1935.

Vulpian was a great friend of Charcot. He was born in Paris of aristocratic descent. His father was a barrister and dramatic author who refused smallpox vaccination, caught the disease and died, leaving his family in dire straits. Vulpian was born just five weeks and two days after Charcot and they were both appointed to the Salpêtrière in 1862 and worked on the section for the aged and the mentally ill. They set about examining all the cases and cataloguing them by diagnosis. Vulpian became more of a laboratory scientist and he beat Charcot in the race to distinction, though the tortoise eventually triumphed over the hare in the fame stakes. Vulpian was made Professor of Pathological Anatomy in 1867 and in 1872 succeeded to the chair of Experimental Pathology leaving the former chair available for Charcot. He was a highly productive scientist writing some 225 scientific papers and he became dean of the medical school. He discovered adrenaline in the medulla (centre) of the adrenal gland above the kidney and was the first to use the term atrial fibrillation for the abnormality of heart rhythm that causes an 'irregularly irregular' pulse. Vulpian died at the age of 61 and Charcot wrote his obituary. A statue to Vulpian was erected in central Paris.

Chapter 6

The Charcot School

Bourneville, Jean-Baptiste Charcot (Charcot's famous son), Gilles de la Tourette, Bouchard, Babinski.

Désiré-Magloire Bourneville (1840-1909)
"A child with a disability has the right to live a full and decent life with dignity…"
UN Convention on *The Rights of the Child*, 1992.
(Bourneville was at least 100 years ahead of the United Nations)

Bourneville was born in Garencières, Normandy. The family firm produced fertiliser from faecal waste. On entering the Paris medical school in 1859 he soon came under the influence of Charcot, an influence that was lifelong, as it was for many. In 1866 he volunteered for work in a cholera epidemic in Amiens and was officially commended by the city authorities. He was one of the first to use a clinical thermometer and his MD thesis in 1870 was on clinical thermometry after cerebral haemorrhage (Wunderlich's classic account of temperature in disease only appeared in 1868 and Clifford Albutt had had his handy short-stemmed mercury thermometers made in Leeds in 1867). The tympanic (ear) thermometer was first described in *JAMA* (*Journal of the American Medical Association*) in 1969 although its use did not become popular until later. Albutt spent time with Duchenne and Trousseau at the Salpêtrière before becoming Regius Professor of Physic in Cambridge in 1892. Bourneville trained with Louis Delasiauve, a pioneer child psychiatrist, epileptologist and advocate for the education of children with learning difficulties, working mainly at the Bicêtre.

In 1879, whilst working as a locum for Delasiauve under Charcot at the Salpêtrière, Bourneville had a patient called Marie. She was 15 years old and from the age of three had had severe learning difficulties, uncontrollable epilepsy and a rash on her face. She died in the hospital and at post mortem examination Bourneville found dense tubers (lumps) in the sulci (grooves) of the cerebral cortex and tumours in the kidneys. He called the condition '*sclerose tubereuse des circonvolutions cerebrales*' (tuberous sclerosis of the cerebral convolutions) but for many years it was known as Bourneville's disease.

Bourneville took charge of the boys' unit at the Bicêtre remaining there until he retired in 1903. He was also a politician, in 1876 he joined the Paris city council and between 1883 and 1889 he was a member of the National Assembly where he promoted the cause of health and social reforms. He was a supporter of Clemenceau and had the ear of Gambetta the head of government. He was a self- professed freethinker and a strong critic of religious influence in public affairs. He wrote about such things as possession and witchcraft, countering them with scientific explanations. He deplored the use of untrained nuns as nurses and was instrumental in introducing secular schools of nursing, first at the Salpêtrière. He was president of the Cremation Society and left instructions for his own cremation. At the Bicêtre he brought in architects to build a new building and bought land with his own money to provide gardens, a gym, an infirmary and play and sports equipment for the children.

Bourneville was passionate about the education of children with learning difficulties, however severe, insisting that no child was beyond help. He teamed up with a former superintendent at the Bicêtre, Hippolyte T Vallée, to establish the Foundation Vallée, a medico-educational institute for such children. It seems anomalous that Bourneville is remembered for describing a single case of tuberous sclerosis and not for the work to which he devoted his life. His wife died in 1906 and Bourneville died, isolated and impoverished, in 1909. He should be remembered as an exceptional and dedicated paediatrician.

Charcot's famous son, Jean-Baptiste-Étienne-Auguste Charcot (1867-1936)

"I must go down to the sea again, to the lonely sea and the sky
And all I ask is a tall ship and a star to steer her by."

John Masefield, 1902.

Charcot's son was born in the house in Neuilly-sur-Seine in 1876. He was a free spirit and didn't fancy a career in medicine but, to please his father, he qualified in Paris and worked with his father at the Salpêtrière, although his real love was

6. The Charcot School

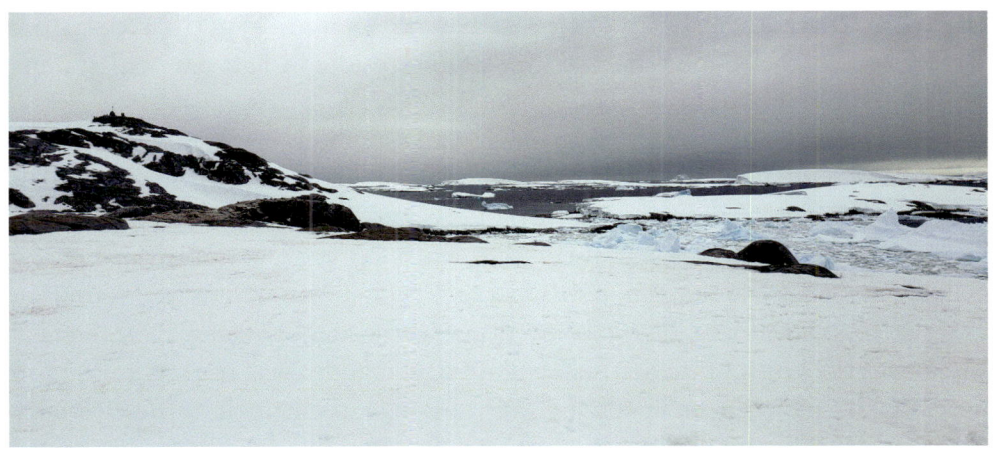

Charcot Bay.

the sea and sailing. In 1893 when the senior Charcot died, Jean-Baptiste inherited a fortune of 400,000 Francs. Soon after, he sailed around the Shetlands, the Hebrides, the Faroes and Iceland in a small schooner. In succession he owned two more boats, the *Francais* and the *Pourquois Pas?* which became recognised as prototype polar vessels. He was a great French patriot and his motivation was his love of the sea, exploration and the honour of his country.

As a scientist and explorer Jean-Baptiste gained enormous public and government support in France and his fame exceeded that of his father. He led the two French Antarctic Expeditions of 1904-07 and 1908-10 mapping the Antarctic coastline and there are at least six places in the Antarctic that carry the Charcot name, the first of which he named after and dedicated to his father,

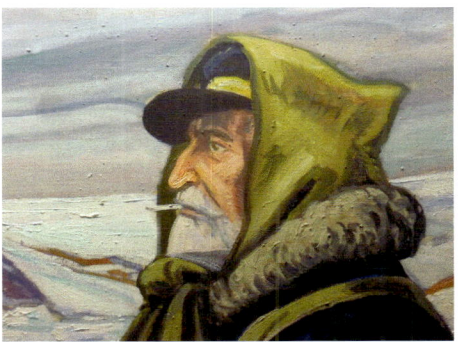

Jean-Baptiste Charcot.

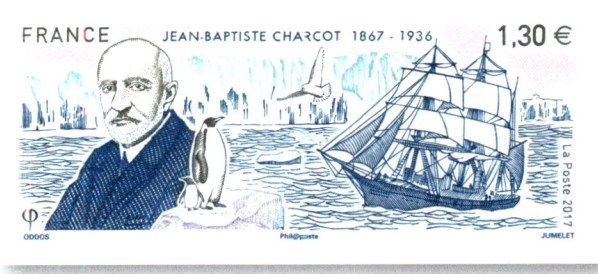

there are: Charcot Bay, Charcot Cove, Charcot Deep Sea Fan, Charcot Island, Port Charcot and Cape Charcot. Both father and son had national stamps issued in their honour.

But his seafaring cost him first a wife and ultimately his life. His first wife was Jeanne Hugo, the granddaughter of Victor Hugo and previously married to Léon Daudet. Daudet and Jean-Baptiste had been good friends but the friendship had ended when they were both up for an internship at the Salpêtrière and Daudet failed while the young Charcot passed, tempting Daudet to suggest that he had only done so through his father's influence. Whatever the truth of that (it seems doubtful, Daudet was never a very good student and gave up on medicine and does not seem to have been a very pleasant man) Jeanne tired of his long absences and divorced him. His second wife, Marguerite was more tolerant and she would accompany him as far as southern Patagonia before turning for home. He was also a sportsman and won two silver medals for sailing in the 1900 Paris Olympics held at the World Fair where Gilles de la Tourette was medical director. He was a very popular man. He knew Captain Scott (Scott of the Antarctic) who referred to him as "the polar gentleman".

He took many other scientists on his expeditions and they added to knowledge about meteorology, tidal systems, atmospherics, gravitation, mineralogy, biology, bacteriology and glaciology. He was elected to scientific societies around the world and given gold medals by the Geographical Societies of Paris, Brussels, Antwerp, London, New York and St. Petersburg.

His life ended tragically at the age of 69 in 1936 when the *Pourquois Pas?* was caught in a storm off the coast of Iceland and went down with only one survivor.

Georges Albert Édouard Brutus Gilles de la Tourette (1857-1904)
"You gave us so much, you promised us more, but then you fell down, at Eros's door."

I can attest that 40 years ago few people had heard of Gilles de la Tourette. Now every astrologer, stable boy and dog walker's apprentice is familiar with the name Tourette. Olivier Walusinski in his very detailed biography explains that this change is in all probability due to an awakening of the appreciation of the intrinsic poetic beauty of the phrase 'Malady of Gilles de la Tourette', itself a consequence of the fortuitous occurrence of an iambus following a

6. The Charcot School

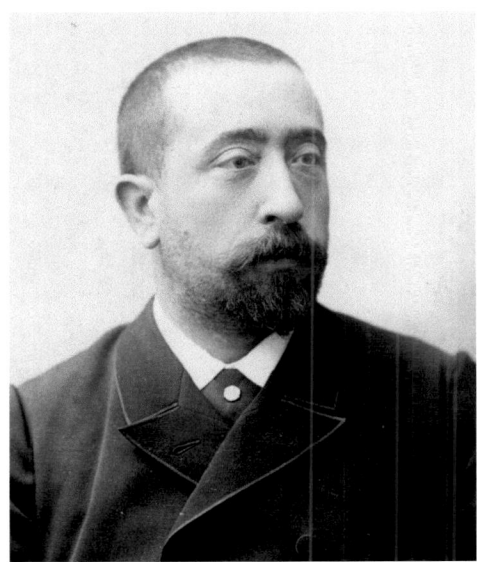

Gilles de la Tourette.

dactyl, as was pointed out to him by MacDonald Critchley, neurologist and biographer of John Hughlings Jackson (see later). An iambus is defined in *Collins English Dictionary* as "a metrical foot consisting of two syllables, a short one followed by a long one, (-_)" or di dah, (Tou-rette) and a dactyl is (-_ _) or di dah dah (Ma-la-dy)." I've put in the dis and dahs because I find them easier than –s and _s. All very academic, learned and correct but (I hesitate to say it of such an eminent physician *but*) I suspect that MacDonald Critchley may have been barking up the *mauvais arbre*. I had believed that Gilles de la Tourette's precipitate rise up the charts was all the result of the vicarious amusement to be had from hearing the sudden explosive use of the word f*****g, or even thinking about hearing the sudden explosive use of the word f*****g (I refer only to the popular concept of the disease). I promise you, the words '*tours d'ivoire*' have never passed my lips, well not in this context.

Gilles de la Tourette was born on 30th October 1857 in the region of Poitou, south of Brittany, in the village of Saint-Gervais not far from the town of Chatelleraut and north of Poitiers. The family name had been Gilles and de la Tourette was added in the 18th century. His parents were a shopkeeper and a housewife but the family had a medical tradition with 12 doctors in four generations. The use of the name Tourette alone was something brought in by an American parents' group because they thought the full surname too much to cope with.

Georges was brilliant at school but when it came to choosing a medical school his mother thought him too young and immature to withstand the rough and tumble of the Parisian Latin Quarter wherein (almost) lies the Salpêtrière. So he was sent first to Poitiers before moving on to Paris. Gilles de la Tourette failed his first exam in Paris on 'Bones in the orbital cavity'. If that question is reported correctly the correct answer would be, "There are no bones in the orbital cavity, it is a cavity, full of eye". Perhaps the question was about the bones that surround and form the orbital cavity. I'd need an atlas of anatomy to answer that one now, though I could have done it with ease sixty odd years ago. Babinski (see next chapter) who was in the same year, being just 18 days younger, passed the exam. Georges' first placement on the wards was to the world's first children's hospital, the Paris *Hôpital des Enfants Malades*, founded in 1802. He was allocated as a student to Charcot at the Salpêtrière in 1884 and he was still a student when in 1885 he wrote the article on *La Maladie des Tics* (the one of the iambus and dactyl after the addition of his name to it) that was to ensure his lasting fame, though that fame was interrupted for many years. Charcot looked after his more capable students and they all but worshipped him, he suggested topics for them to look into, monitored their progress, encouraged when necessary, praised when appropriate and promoted their work on completion. Georges was in awe of 'the Master' (who wasn't?) and remained a devoted disciple for the rest of his short life. He became Charcot's chef de Clinique, equivalent to the English senior registrar in my day. He organised the department and attended the high society evenings at Charcot's home where he met several notables including Sigmund Freud.

Freud came to the Salpêtrière for four months in 1885-86 and fell under the Charcot spell, so much so that he named his first son Jean-Martin. Charcot could do no wrong and Freud wrote to his wife to say how much he was enjoying and benefiting from his time with him. After Charcot died Freud wrote "The glory of Charcot will always stand above the opinions of his time". I'm not sure what that means, possibly that Freud thought that Charcot wasn't sufficiently appreciated during his lifetime, but it's a bit of a two-handed compliment. Jeffrey Lieberman, a prominent American psychiatrist and former president of the American Psychiatric Association, refers to Freud in his 2015 book *Shrinks* as "simultaneously psychiatry's greatest hero and it's most calamitous fraud". He relates how Freud was a dictator who would excommunicate from his close circle of friends and fellow believers those who questioned his theories (not a scientist then), but was also perceptive in many ways. Peter Medawar (1915-87) a Nobel laureate, one of the founders of the science of immunology and one of the sharpest of scientific minds, wrote in his 1982 book *Pluto's Republic* "Psychoanalytic theory is the most stupendous intellectual confidence trick of the 20th century". No shilly-shallying there then. Gilles de la Tourette progressed in the hierarchy at the Salpêtrière becoming *Médecins des Hôpitaux* (consultant) and competing for a professorship but never quite achieving it. He had a talent for writing and wrote prolifically on neurological topics. And then disaster struck.

1893

The year 1893 for Gilles de la Tourette has often been described as his *annus horribilis*. It was not an annus horribilis, by any reasonable standard it was an *annus horribilissimus* of the kind that probably few of us could come through unscathed. In July his five year old son Jean (was he too named after Charcot?) died of meningitis. Six weeks later in August, the man he admired more than any other, his beloved Charcot, died at the age of 67 of coronary disease with acute left ventricular failure while on the way to Burgundy for a holiday. But there was still more to come. The final knife to be plunged into his heart came that December, when a former patient tried to murder him. On the evening of 6 December 1893 Gilles de la Tourette was at home when a 29-year old woman, Mrs. Rose Kamper, came and insisted on seeing him. She said that she had been hypnotised by several doctors, one of them Gilles de la Tourette, and the result was that her personality had been so affected she was no longer able to earn a living and was destitute. Gilles de la Tourette promised to do what he could to find aid for her and turned to the door when she pulled out a gun and fired three shots. The first shot glanced off the back of his skull (occipital bone) finishing up about two inches from the point of entry, between skin and bone (perhaps bullet speed was less in those days?). The next two were later found in the furniture.

Gilles de la Tourette was soon relieved of his bullet and recovered from his physical injury over the next few days. But from then on his mental condition deteriorated. His behaviour would at times be comically absurd, though clearly

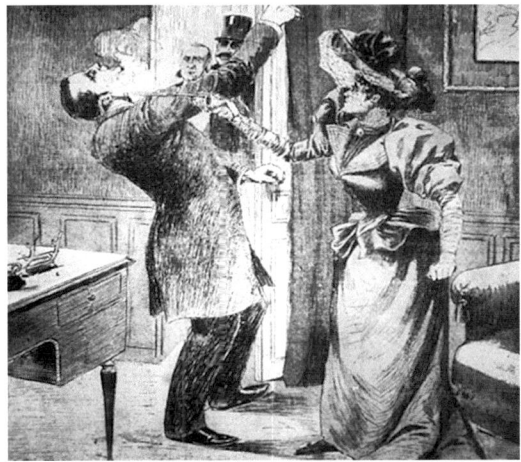

1893 depiction of the shooting of Gilles de la Tourette.

alarming. On asking an examination candidate who were the three greatest French physicians of the 19th century and being told, Laennec, Duchenne and Charcot, he rubbished the student, claiming that the correct answer was "My [Gilles de la Tourette's] grandfather, my father and me." The date of that incident is not recorded, but his first public howler was not until 1901. He had agreed to give an introductory talk at the theatre to a new play about a woman who had slept, or gone into a lethargic state, for six years after a "terrible fright". Gilles de la Tourette's talk was to be about pathological sleep states, but he rambled on endlessly until the audience resorted to jeers and catcalls.

He went on to develop delusions of grandeur as a symptom of general paralysis of the insane (GPI), brain infection with syphilis, though neither Charcot nor Gilles de la Tourette ever accepted its syphilitic basis. In December 1902 a court, following a submission by the family, agreed that he could no longer manage his affairs and a guardian chosen by the family was appointed. He died in an asylum in Switzerland, the terminal event being a prolonged epileptic fit (status epilepticus) a known complication of GPI. There seems little to doubt about the clinical diagnosis of GPI but not much has been made in diagnostic terms of his *annus horribilissimus*. He must surely have suffered great stress that year and stress was often mentioned as an aggravating factor for GPI. Whether he ever displayed the recognised diagnostic features of post-traumatic stress disorder (PTSD), I think we cannot know, but it is often said that he deteriorated noticeably after the terrible events of that year and it seems possible, or even probable, that they played a part in his downfall.

GPI has been seen very rarely since the discovery of penicillin, or perhaps not at all in recent years. There has though been an increase in syphilis in the UK in recent years; in 2019, 7,982 cases were recorded, an increase of 10% since 2018. Possibly, the rate will have fallen in 2020 as a consequence of the lockdowns. A much more famous contemporary who died in an asylum was Vincent van Gogh (1853-1890). It was suggested that he too may have had GPI but the suggestion has been rejected, largely on the grounds that not enough time had passed between his possible exposure to syphilis in the brothels of Paris and his becoming mentally ill. A whole string of alternative psychiatric diagnoses has been proposed. If you visit the St. Paul asylum, now at least in part, Clinique Van Gogh in St. Rémy de Provence where van Gogh died (admittedly one of the lesser reasons to visit Provence) you can see his medical documents and his room with the famous chair that he painted in 1888. If I remember correctly the hospital now specialises in art and music therapy. I have a mental picture of Gilles de la Tourette as a sad Van Gogh-like figure adrift in a sea of brilliant neurologists (I include neurosurgeons and neuropathologists): Charcot, Babinski, Marie, Brown-Séquard, Hughlings Jackson, Broca, Horsley, Alzheimer, Gowers, though had he lived long enough he might have proved himself one of their company.

If you survey people of all ages around the world about 1 in 2,000 will have Tourette syndrome but if you confine your survey to children it will approach 1%. The tics are either motor (usually rapid twitches) or vocal (noises). Simple motor tics (blinking, shrugging, grimacing) usually begin at around the age of seven and more complex motor tics (jumping, squatting, licking, smelling) a few years later. Simple vocal tics (throat clearing, grunting, sniffing, snorting) may start at about 11, and complex vocal tics, such as coprolalia (literally, faecal speech) from the age of 15, but they are much less common. Symptoms of Attention Deficit Hyperactivity Disorder (ADHD) or Obsessive Compulsive Disorder (OCD) commonly occur together with Tourette syndrome. Many people seem to improve or recover completely in late adolescence or early adult life but they may be prone to recurrence later at times of stress.

Perhaps the most famous sufferer from Tourette syndrome was the great Dr. Samuel Johnson of Lichfield, who was prone to making multiple whistles and other noises together with unusual mannerisms. In his dictionary he defines a swearer as, "A wretch who obtests the great name wantonly and profanely". I know nothing about the verb to obtest, other than that he defines it as, "To beseech; to supplicate" and quotes Dryden, "Suppliants demand, a truce with olive branches in their hand, obtest his clemency, and from the plain, beg leave to draw the bodies of their slain."

Mozart was apparently a funny chap and may or may not have had Tourette syndrome. There was also an aristocratic socialite, a marchioness no less, the Marquise de Dampierre, described in the early 19th century by a physician called Jean-Gaspard Itard and given to coprolalia. She had suffered from the condition since the age of seven, progressing as described from simple motor tics to complex motor tics, through simple vocal tics to complex vocal tics and coprolalia. She was never a patient of Charcot but in one of his lectures he told of passing her on the stairs at a social gathering and in the short period they were in transit he heard her say "s**t" and "f*****g pigs", presumably *"Merde"* and "*Putain de cochon*", thus staying true to the origins of the word coprolalia (Greek, again, from *kopros*, dung, faeces, or s**t, and *lalein,* to babble).

Today there are special clinics for Tourette syndrome. Diagnostic criteria include both motor and vocal tips, several times a day either continuously or intermittently, beginning before the age of 18 changing over time and not due to medication. Such clinics may see a hundred or more patients a year usually drawing from a large area. It's obviously a very serious business despite the hilarity. The patients can't help it and those with severe disease are much embarrassed and socially, educationally and occupationally disabled. It says much for Gilles de la Tourette that he recognised the problem. I've read that Tourette symptoms have increased in young people during the pandemic (could that be one result of the increased publicity given to the syndrome in recent years?).

Charles Bouchard (1837-1915)
Antagonist of Charcot and denier of Babinski

Bouchard was born in the small town of Montier-en-Der in the Haute Marne department of north east France, about 150 miles from Paris. He studied medicine first in Lyon and then in Paris under Charcot and graduated MD in 1866 with a thesis on aneurysms of the cerebral circulation as causes of brain haemorrhage. He rose rapidly through the hierarchy, becoming a full professor in 1879 after he had been appointed physician to the Bicêtre in 1874. After being trained by Charcot and writing papers with him, he apparently became a rival of his previous mentor and things came to a head most notably over the *agrégation* examinations of Babinski in 1892 (see later).

Bouchard's name is attached to Bouchard's nodes, bony excrescences at the proximal finger joints (the ones nearer the wrist) seen in osteoarthritis. In the 18th century the English physician William Heberden had described similar bony swellings in the distal finger joints (nearer the nails) in the same disease. Bouchard's nodes seem indistinguishable from Heberden's nodes apart from being in adjacent joints and the newer eponym seems superfluous. Bouchard attracted much criticism especially from the friends of Charcot. In 1887 he made a speech in which he paid extravagant compliments to Charcot and proclaimed the debt he owed to him. It was widely condemned as hypocritical but Guillain (a later occupant of Charcot's chair of neurology, see later) insisted that the repentance was sincere, although late in the day.

Joseph Jules François Félix Babinski (1857-1932)

"With this sign shall you prevail."

The Emperor Constantine (288-337AD).

Charcot's greatest pupil

Joseph Babinski was born in Paris on 12 November 1857 to Aleksander Babinski and Henryeta Weren Babinska, a Polish couple who had fled Poland during Russian repressions in 1848. Aleksander was a "professional revolutionary", almost a prototype Che Guevara (I once met Che's daughter, she is a paediatrician in Cuba, where Che is idolised). He had participated in several uprisings against the Russians before fleeing Poland. He was an inconstant father to Joseph and his elder brother, Henri and husband to Henryeta. He returned to Poland to support a new insurrection in 1863 showing up again to his wife and children in Paris in 1871, then being involved in

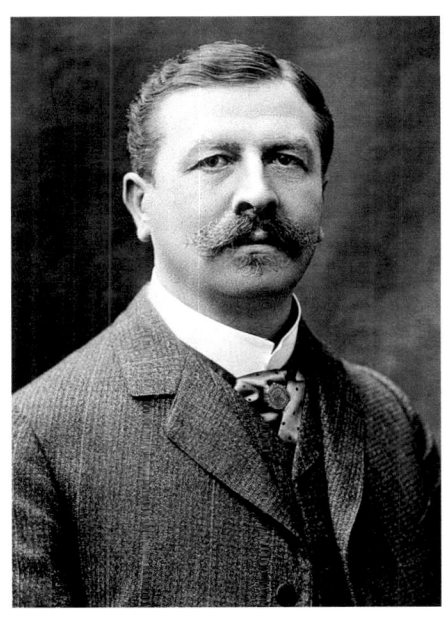

Joseph Babinski.

the Paris Commune of that year that led to the establishment of the 3rd Republic after Napoleon III had been captured in the Franco-Prussian war the previous year. Aleksander's final escapade involved being temporarily exiled from France in 1874 and distinguishing himself as an engineer in Peru where he was made a freeman of the country during a war between Peru and Chile. The city of Lima has a Babinski garden, a Babinski museum and a Babinski memorial. He returned to Paris in 1887 and died in 1899 in the apartment he shared with Joseph, so clearly the father and son relationship was not destroyed by his frequent absences. Henryeta is described as a well-educated woman who for several years was a private tutor to a well-known family. Her two sons loved and respected her.

The two brothers attended the Polish school in Paris and grew up to be both French and Polish patriots. Henri was two years older than Joseph and perhaps of a less serious disposition. He trained as a mining engineer and worked for a time in French Guyana pointing to the finding of rich gold deposits. On a similar quest in Patagonia he found no gold but extensive seams of coal. He achieved fame, though, as a gourmet with the pseudonym Ali-Bab and had a body shape to prove his interest in food. His book *Gastronomie Pratique* is, so I'm told, still regarded as a culinary classic. The origin of the pseudonym is disputed, but to those of us who enjoyed the pantomimes as children it seems fairly obvious.

The two brothers lived together for many years and were regarded as inseparable. They had changed their names from Henryk and Jozef to Henri and Joseph. Nothing is known of Babinski's personal life but Leon Babinski, a distant relative and self-proclaimed friend, claimed that 'Jozef' had three daughters 'born out of wedlock' to a Norwegian mother living close to Paris, and went on to mention Henryk and 'a lady of his heart' who attended Jozef's funeral. Whether Babinski ever acknowledged or supported his daughters, or whether they existed, I don't know. He was described as a tall handsome man of attractive bearing and a usually silent disposition. He and Charcot shared a habit of retreating into lengthy silent contemplation during the examination of a patient.

Joseph Babinski attended the medical school in Paris and worked his way through the many and acknowledgedly tough exams and the junior medical ranks. He had graduated in 1885 with a thesis on 'An anatomical and clinical study of multiple sclerosis'. He became *chef de service* to Charcot later in 1885 by way of a tragedy when the incumbent died and he remained close to Charcot until the latter's death in 1893. In 1890 he made his fifth annual attempt at the examination for the title of *médecins des Hôpitaux* in which he had previously got high marks but been pipped at the post each time, because of the very few out of many candidates who were allowed through. This time he made it. The next and final exam, and the gateway to a professorship, was the *Agrégation de Médecins* exam which he took in 1892 and which led to the granddaddy of medical academic hoo-has. There was a panel of nine examiners, all appointed by the Minister for Education and 16 candidates of whom five would be successful. The senior examiner was Professor Charles Bouchard, former pupil and present enemy of Charcot, who it seems, was not beyond a little wrangling and arranging things to his own advantage, or so it was alleged. When the results of the prolonged written and clinical examinations were published, four out of the five known 'Bouchard men' got through and the two known 'Charcot men' including Babinski were dumped. There followed two years of heated argument and Babinski and four other unsuccessful candidates made a formal complaint to the minister. There was a row in the press with some newspapers supporting the complainers and some the examiners. The British Medical Journal poked its nose into private French misery with an article pointing to the iniquities of the exam and the future French Prime Minister, Georges Clemenceau, wrote a newspaper article demanding that the exam results be pronounced null and void. In classical political style the matter was shelved for two years until, in 1894, the *Conseil d'État* pronounced the exams legal and valid and that was the end of it. Babinski gave up on an academic career and never bothered with the exam again. It has been suggested, perhaps by Babinski himself, that failing the exam was good for his career because it freed him from the administrative duties of a professor and allowed him to concentrate on his clinical and research work. But being a professor hadn't noticeably hindered Charcot, or Bouchard, and Babinski was certainly of professorial calibre.

Babinski was not the only one to develop a strong dislike for Bouchard. Léon Daudet, a well-known journalist and novelist of the time and friend of the Charcot family, didn't hold back. He wrote of Bouchard, "He gives to the observer the impression of unbelievable stupidity coupled with tremendous self-satisfaction." He also threw in, "metaphysicist, fanciful clinician, ignorant creator of diseases, sad, full of bitterness, a dull voice, and a suspicious look", just to make sure he'd made his point, which of course makes us wonder about Daudet and think that perhaps Bouchard wasn't so bad a chap after all. Bouchard did have friends and later in his life he paid fulsome tribute to Charcot, which may or may not have been accepted at face value (I think it usually wasn't).

Léon Daudet (1867-1942) appears to have been an exceptionally vituperative and virulent man. The son of a famous novelist, Alphonse Daudet, he was a medical student at the Salpêtrière but never qualified and then went into journalism and wrote novels. In addition to writing over-the-top outrageous criticisms he founded a very right wing newspaper, campaigned as a monarchist and anti-democrat, and supported the Vichy government of Marshall Petain (I suppose every good story has a villain). He knew Charcot well, despite having previously broken off a friendship with Charcot's son, and was present when Charcot had his first episode of severe cardiac pain in 1891.

It was at Charcot's home late at night after a meal and Pasteur was also present. Professor Potain, the cardiologist, who with Charcot had cared for Duchenne at the end of his life, lived nearby and was roused from his bed. He reassured Charcot but in a whisper to others predicted that he would last only another two and a half years. He proved disturbingly accurate.

The French medical exams system of those days seems to have been tough almost to the extent of cruelty, in the attempt to find the 'elite'. The entrant to French medicine had to face exams for the externship, then the internship, and then present a thesis for the MD when, if successful, he became qualified to pursue a career outside hospital. If he (there were no women) then wanted to proceed in hospital he would take the exams for *médecins des hôpitaux* and finally, to reach the highest level, the *agrégation de médecine* after which he could become a professor, but it wasn't guaranteed. All the exams were competitive with only a set number getting through, so even if you did very well you could still fail and often did, according to the roll of the dice or the machinations of men. I gather that the French system has changed greatly since Babinski's day with the abolition of the separation between hospital and university and the simplification of the exam system making life much less complicated for undergraduate and postgraduate students.

For a year from 1894 Babinski was in charge of a fever hospital but in 1895 he became Head of Internal Medicine at the Pitié Hospital which had been founded in 1612 by Marie de Medici, the wife and widow of Henry IV, the assassinated king, and mother and regent of Louis XIII. Babinski stayed at the Pitié until 1922 (for 27 years) until he had to retire at the age of 65. He continued his private practice for another seven years. The Pitié was a run-down hospital described as a "cadaverous worm-eaten tomb", and it was deliberately and officially burned down in 1912. The following year the new Pitié, on a site near the Salpêtrière, was opened by President of France, Poincaré. It was combined with the Salpêtrière as the Pitié-Salpêtrière in 1964.

Babinski developed a great reputation at the Pitié as a neurologist and a teacher and, like Charcot, attracted doctors from far and wide as either students or co-workers. He taught on case studies on Saturday mornings and although a neurologist, he retained his competence in general internal medicine. He always paid great respect to Charcot. At that time hospital physicians were paid only a token salary which had to be added to by private practice, which in Babinski's case became very large and lucrative. He became the neurologist to Parisian high society, counting among his patients such people as Marcel Proust, Marshall Petain, and the King of Spain and his fees reflected that fact. Proust was bewildered when Babinski asked him to repeat the words *constantinopolitain* and *artilleur del'artilerie,* looking presumably, for signs of dysarthria (an inability to articulate properly because of weakness or incoordination of the muscles of speech). The most common cause of dysarthria is alcohol intoxication but it can be the result of neurological disease. It is to be distinguished from dysphasia which is an inability to form or find words, or the correct words, because of disease of the brain often after a stroke. In my day the usual tests for dysarthria were, 'the Leith Police dismisseth us', 'the Royal Ulster Constabulary' and 'the Irish (or was it Hibernian?) Fusiliers'. Proust's comment was, "When the most skilful professor tells you to pronounce [those words] you do not know what the significance of it may be and he himself believes that you do not know."

Babinski's sign

Babinski first described his sign at the Biological Society of Paris on 22 February 1896, his description is said to have consisted of 28 lines, although in book form it's less than that. In it he refers to a 'pinprick' of the sole of the foot causing 'extension of the toes on the metatarsus on the paralysed side', in cases of hemiplegia. In this account Babinki described a flexion of the whole leg on both the normal and the paralysed side and refers to extension of the 'toes', not just the big toe, on the paralysed side. He later added fanning of the toes as an associated phenomenon. He initially developed the sign to distinguish between an organic and a 'hysterical' paralysis.

For an explanation of Babinski's sign for non-medical readers see the Addendum at the end of this chapter.

Babinski developed a large reputation to rival that of Charcot and was much honoured posthumously, especially in Poland. At one time he was proposed by professors at a Polish university for a Nobel Prize. His greatest memorial, however, is the Babinski Building at the Salpêtrière. Finished in 1996, it includes an Institute of Myology (the study of muscle), the Babinski lecture hall, and the departments of neurosurgery, neuroradiology, ophthalmology and ear, nose and throat surgery.

Never a surgeon, Babinski played a large part in the birth of French neurosurgery. Towards the end of the 19th century neurosurgery consisted almost entirely of the removal of a few brain tumours and the results, by and large, were dismal although there had been limited success in the treatment of focal epilepsy. The first neurosurgery journal appeared in France soon after Babinski started at the Pitié in 1895. He became interested in trying to locate brain and spinal cord lesions, mainly the latter, with enough precision to allow surgery to be successful (there was no imaging to guide the process). He became confident enough to refer a patient with a spinal tumour to Victor Horsley, the great pioneer of British neurosurgery in London (I don't know the result). With brain tumours, Babinski hung on for many years lacking confidence in the results, though he did refer some patients for operation to decompress the brain.

Babinski saw the potential of neurosurgery and was a great and early advocate for it. He first collaborated with a surgeon called Thierry de Martel who, as a general surgeon, considered himself insufficiently trained in neurology but was a friend of Clovis Vincent who had trained in neurology at the Salpêtrière. De Martel and Vincent became France's great neurosurgical double act, the one teaching the other surgery and the other teaching that one neurology. They were lucky that Vincent had the surgical skills. De Martel had been to London to learn from Horsley. On his deathbed in 1932 Babinski was asked what had given him the greatest satisfaction, he didn't say 'the sign', instead he said, "showing the way to neurosurgery to de Martel and Vincent." He would attend neurosurgical operations to see what was going on and to advise about the neurology. At a Neurological Society meeting in 1928 de Martel described Babinski as "the first supporter of neurosurgery in France and our leader". Clearly that is why the building that now houses the department of neurosurgery at the Salpêtrière is called the Babinski building.

Babinski died on 29 October 1932. He had been suffering from Parkinson's disease for several years, as had his father before him and was

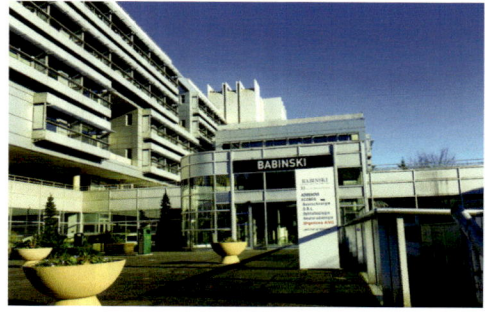

Babinski building.

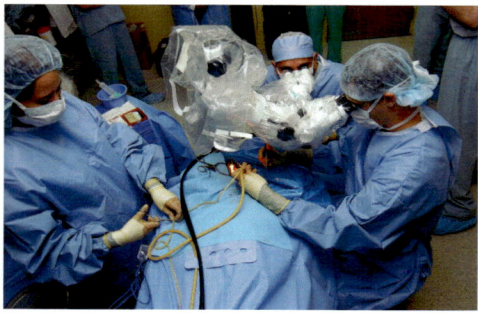

Neurosurgery.

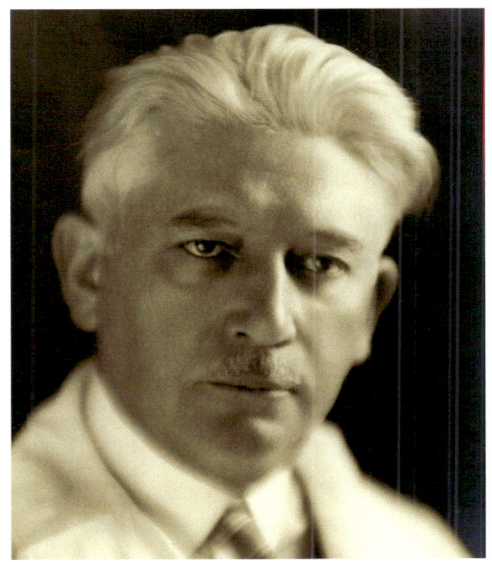
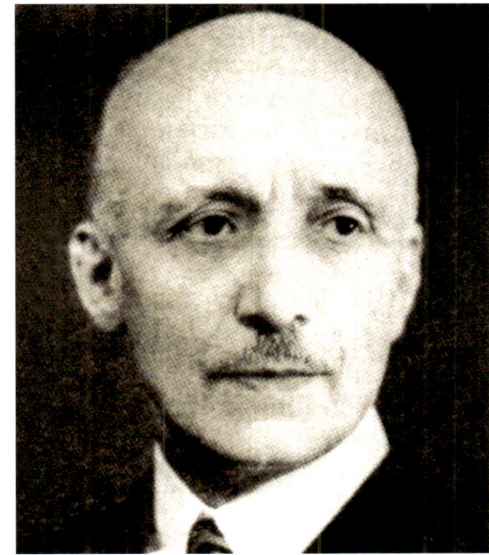

Clovis Vincent. *Thierry de Martel.*

deeply affected by the death of his brother the previous year. He was entombed alongside his parents and his brother in the Polish cemetery in Montmorency in the northern suburbs of Paris.

The final paragraph of Philippon and Poirier's biography states: "Joseph Babinski, this blue-eyed, good-looking giant, was not a genius nor a god, but a man, a great man – at the same time a great clinician and great consultant, a great Frenchman and a great Pole. Why should he not be recognised for eternity *as just a man, as every man, equal to all and better than none?*" (my italics). That last part is itself a quotation from Jean-Paul Sartre. Five greats in a single sentence and then finishing up as just one of the throng seems more than a little contrarian.

Addendum for non-medical readers

An explanation of Babinski's sign

Babinski's sign indicates a positive result of Babinski's test, the purpose of which, will become clear. The test is performed by taking a sharp(ish) tool, most patella hammers for testing knee and ankle jerks have a pointed end for this purpose or car keys may do the job. The pointed end is scraped along the sole of the foot beginning at the outside of the heel and moving along the outside of the sole and then along the base of the toes to the base of the big toe. You watch the big toe. Normally it should move downwards, towards the ground or away from the body. That is a normal, or flexor, response, a negative test. If the big toe moves upwards, or towards the body, that is an abnormal or extensor response and a positive test (Babinski's sign).

To understand the significance of the test you have to know some basic neuroanatomy. Nerve cells are called neurons (or neurones). Each neuron consists of a cell body with a nucleus, short receptive projections called dendrites where the incoming nerve impulses are received, and a usually long thin projection called the axon that carries the outgoing impulses. When you decide to move your toe the process begins in nerve cells in the brain and the electrical impulse travels down their axons to nerve cells in the spinal cord. There, those brain cell axons meet up with the dendrites of spinal cord neurons at meeting places called synapses where the impulse passes from brain neuron to spinal cord neuron. It then passes down the axon of that neuron within the peripheral nerve to the toe muscles causing them to contract. So it's a two-phase process, brain to spine then spine to muscle. The brain-to-spine neuron is called the 'upper motor neuron' and the spine-to-muscle neuron is the 'lower motor neuron'. Failure of the muscle to respond may be due to a problem at either of the sites (or in the muscle itself) and we speak of upper motor neuron or lower motor neuron paralysis. What Babinski showed is that a positive test is indicative of an upper motor neuron problem. The total of upper motor neurons is called the pyramidal tracts. In young babies, before their pyramidal tracts are fully developed, a positive Babinski sign is normal.

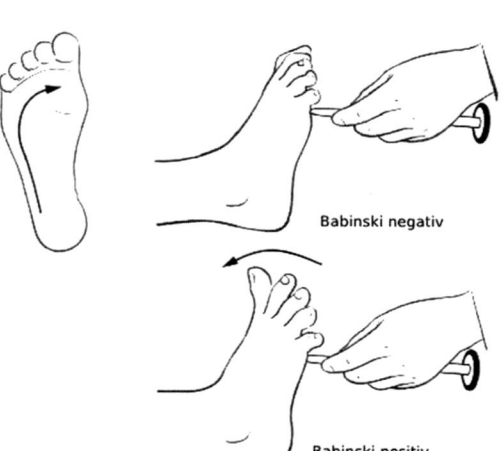

Above: Patella hammer.
Left: Babinski reflex.

Chapter 7

After Charcot

Charcot's successors: Brissaud, Raymond, Dejerine and Klumpke (Madame Dejerine).

"A professor is a gentleman who has a different opinion."
August Bier (1861-1949).

"We know the human brain is a device to keep the ears from grating on one another."
Peter De Vries (1910-1993).

After Charcot, the professors of neurology at the Salpêtrière were Fulgence Raymond from 1894 to 1910, Joseph Dejerine from 1911 to 1917, Pierre Marie from 1917 to 1923 and Georges Guillain from 1923 to 1947. Charcot was an impossible act to follow and while they were thinking about it Edouard Brissaud was appointed as stopgap for a year.

Édouard Brissaud (1852-1909), Temporary Professor 1893-1894

"It is hard to tell how we will eventually understand the brain."
Matthew Cobb, *The Idea of the Brain*, 2020.

Brissaud's career began as an extern with Charcot in 1875 and continued with Charcot until he (Charcot) died. He was said to be Charcot's favourite pupil (there were several contenders for that title including Babinski). Brissaud was born in 1852 in Besancon in eastern France, near the Swiss border, into a distinguished family of artists, musicians and intellectuals. He held in succession the chairs of the History of Medicine and of Medical Pathology.

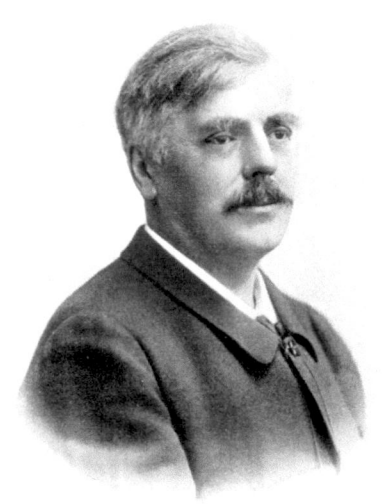

Édouard Brissaud.

There seems to have been a fairly regular progression in professorships: medical history, medical pathology and then whatever was your true *métier*. He was the first to point to the substantia nigra, a mass of pigmented nerve cells in the mid-brain, one of the basal ganglia of the brain, as the seat of Parkinson's disease. He was also a popular teacher and wit, keeping students amused as well as instructed. He was the inspiration for Proust's Dr. du Boulbon in *À la recherche du temps perdue*. He treated Proust for asthma (at that time asthma was thought to have its origins in the nervous system). In the novel, apparently, Dr. du Boulbon is described as "a specialist of nervous diseases, the one whom Charcot, before dying, had said that he would dominate neurology and psychiatry". With Charcot and Marie, Brissaud founded the journal *Revue Neurologique* and he wrote a handbook, *Traité de Médicine*. He died of a brain tumour in 1909 at the age of 57.

Fulgence Raymond (1844-1910), Professor 1894-1910

"The best doctor in the world is the veterinarian. He can't ask his patients what is the matter – he's got to just know."
           Will Rogers (1879-1935).

Raymond was originally a vet but switched to medicine. He worked alongside Babinski and Marie as junior doctors and as professor published research on poliomyelitis, syringomyelia and tabes dorsalis.

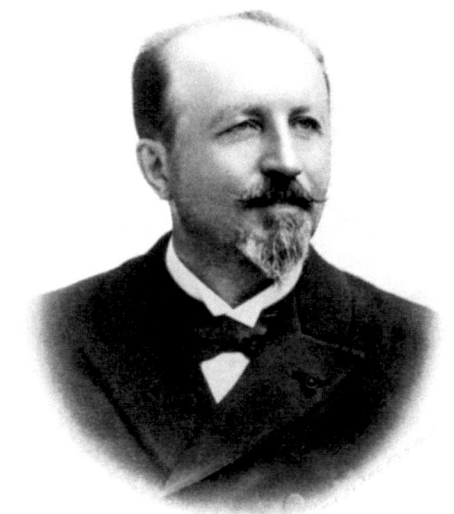

Fulgence Raymond.

Joseph Dejerine (1849-1917), Professor 1911-1917

"The Brain: an apparatus with which we think we think."
    Ambrose Bierce (1842-1914).

Joseph Dejerine, the third professor of neurology at the Salpêtrière, took over in 1911. He had trained in Paris with Alfred Vulpian the discoverer of adrenaline. Dejerine worked initially at the Bicêtre, establishing a pathology laboratory before moving to the Salpêtrière and occupying in succession the chairs of medical history and then of neurology, making many contributions to the study of diseases of the brain. He died of kidney failure in 1917 allowing Marie, at the age of 64, finally to take the chair he had wanted since the death of Charcot.

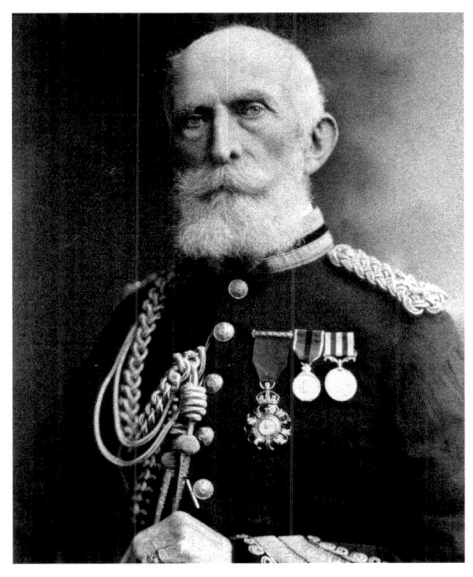

Joseph Dejerine.

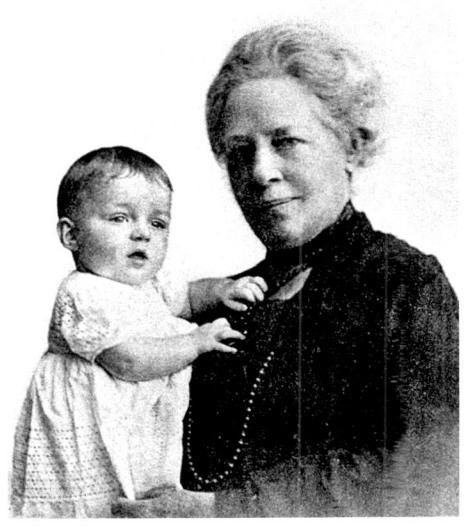

Augusta Marie Dejerine-Klumpke.

Augusta Marie Dejerine-Klumpke (1859-1927)

"Anything you can do I can do better, I can do anything better than you. No you can't. Yes I can. No you can't. Yes I can. No you can't. Yes I can, yes I can, yes I can."
    Irving Berlin, *Annie Get Your Gun*, 1946.

Augusta Marie Klumpke, or Dejerine-Klumpke, the wife of Joseph Dejerine is remembered in paediatrics for Klumpke's palsy, or Dejerine-Klumpke's palsy, the equivalent of Erb-Duchenne palsy but affecting the lower part of the brachial plexus rather than the upper. It may occur after a breech delivery when the baby's arm gets stuck up alongside the head causing stretching of the armpit region and damage to the lower part of the brachial plexus. Augusta was a star in her own right. Born in San Francisco, she was one of the first women to hit the Paris medical scene. She became a prominent neurologist and neuroanatomist and the first woman president of the French Society of Neurology.

Chapter 8

Perpetuating the Fame

Marie, Guillain and Barré

Pierre Marie (1853-1940), Professor 1917-1923

Ambition long frustrated.

Pierre Marie was born in Paris to wealthy parents. His father had wanted him to go into the law but he decided on medicine. He studied in Paris and qualified MD in 1883 with a dissertation on Basedow's disease, which is the continental name for what is known in the UK as Graves' disease, thyrotoxicosis or exophthalmic goitre. He concentrated on the tremor of the hands in that disease, as might be expected of a future professor of neurology.

He had studied with Charcot from 1878 and became *medicin des Hôpitaux* in 1888. In 1886 he had written about, and introduced, the term acromegaly, leading some to claim that he was one of the first endocrinologists, but Marie at that time was unaware that it had anything to do with the pituitary gland or of the existence of hormones. In 1887 the Lithuanian physician Minkowski showed that people with acromegaly had an enlarged pituitary gland at autopsy and by the end of the century it was established that acromegaly was associated with a pituitary tumour. Horsley in London performed successful pituitary surgery beginning in 1904 but it

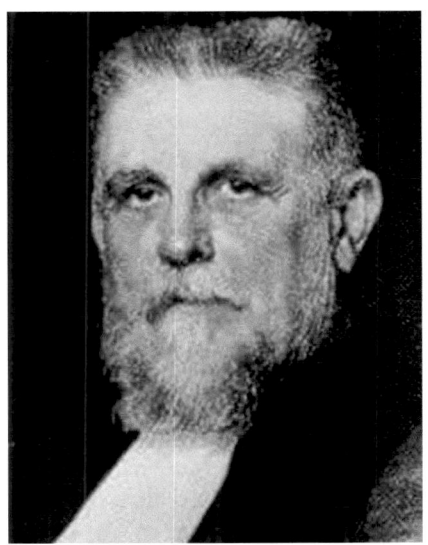

Pierre Marie.

was not until 1945 that the Chinese American chemist Choh Hao Li isolated and analysed growth hormone. At one time acromegaly was known as Marie's disease. In 1893 he described hereditary cerebellar ataxia.

Marie was finally appointed to Charcot's chair of neurology at the age of 64 after the death of Dejerine.

Charcot-Marie-Tooth Disease

In 1886 Charcot and Marie wrote about, 'a particular form of progressive muscular atrophy…' and in the same year Howard Henry Tooth submitted his MD thesis on the same subject. The disease is called Charcot-Marie-Tooth disease. I don't know whether Charcot and Marie ever met Tooth or whether they lie together in medical history as strangers.

Tooth (1856-1925) was born in Hove near Brighton and qualified in medicine at St. Bartholomew's Hospital, London (Bart's). He was appointed to the London Metropolitan Hospital in 1887, to St. Bartholomew's in 1895 and to the National Hospital Queen Square in 1907. The London Metropolitan Hospital was founded in 1836 as a hospital for the poor and needy. Over almost a century and a half it had several closures and relocations until it finally closed in 1977 and the remaining patients were transferred to Bart's. Tooth had a distinguished career both as a doctor and as a soldier. He served in the army for many years rising to the rank of Colonel in the Boer War. Charcot-Marie-Tooth disease is a sensory-motor neuropathy (it affects both the nerves responsible for sensation and those responsible for muscle movement). There are many different genetic subtypes which need to be differentiated by DNA analysis. It begins in childhood and is the most common diagnosis made in a clinic for children with neuromuscular problems. It is slowly progressive but does not usually shorten life expectancy.

Georges Guillain (1876-1961), Professor 1923-1947

"If the war didn't happen to kill you it was bound to start you thinking."
George Orwell.

The first thing to get right about Guillain is how to say his name. For many years I and most other English doctors said 'Ghee Yan' or 'zhee yan' but in 1977 an American doctor who had worked with Guillain wrote a letter to the Journal of the American Medical Association to explain that Guillain said 'Ghee Lan'.

8. Perpetuating the Fame

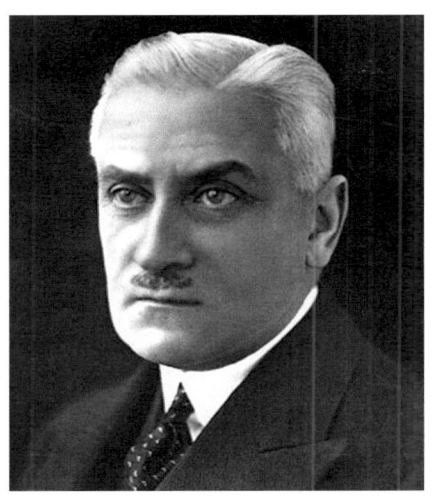

Georges Guillain.

Georges Guillain was born in Rouen, into a well-off family. His father was an engineer and his mother the daughter of a wealthy industrialist. He studied medicine in Rouen for two years and then transferred to Paris. In 1898 as a student he wrote about disorders of the brachial plexus. He graduated MD in 1902 with a dissertation on syringomyelia, a condition in which a cyst develops in the middle of the spinal cord, usually secondary to a malformation at the base of the brain. He passed the *agrégation* exam in 1910. During the First World War he was head of neurology in the French 6th army. There he met up with Jean Barré, they worked together and formed a lifelong friendship. It was at that time that they examined two soldiers who within a short time of each other developed a condition that was previously unknown. It was a polyneuropathy (a condition affecting many of the nerves in the body) and they showed that its peculiarity was what they called *"disassociation cyto-albuminique"* cell-protein disassociation in the cerebrospinal fluid (CSF, the fluid that surrounds and protects the brain and spinal cord and is obtained by lumbar puncture). With cell-protein disassociation there is a high level of protein in the CSF but no increase in cells such as is found in meningitis. It is characteristic of Guillain-Barré syndrome. The name Guillain-Barré syndrome was not applied until 1927. The name of Strohl, the electrophysiologist who did electrical measurements on the patients was added (Guillain-Barré-Strohl syndrome) but people usually stick to the double name.

After the war Guillain worked at the Charité Hôpital in Paris, another hospital that began with Marie de Medici in the 17th century. Those buildings were pulled down in 1935 and replaced by the new Paris Faculty of Medicine. He was appointed to the chair of neurology at the Salpêtrière to follow Marie in 1923 and remained in that post until 1947 when he retired. He received many honours including Commander of the *Légion d'Honneur*. Together with Barré in 1920 he wrote a book about their work in the war and he later wrote a biography of Charcot. He died in Paris in 1961.

Jean Alexandre Barré (1880-1967)

Barré was born and received his medical education in Nantes, a city in the Western Loire, south of Brittany and over 200 miles from Paris. After qualifying he moved to Paris to work with Babinski. In 1912 he published a thesis on the joint disease associated with tabes dorsalis (Charcot's joint). He met Guillain during the war when they collaborated on the Guillain-Barré syndrome. It is said that he published over 800 papers (I wonder, that seems an incredible number). He was appointed professor of neurology in Strasbourg in 1919 and developed a particular expertise in the neurology of the inner ear and the functioning of the balance mechanism there. He founded a journal on 'oto-neuro-ophthalmology'. At the age of 73 (presumably he was long retired) he had a stroke which left him paralysed down one side but he was still able to attend medical meetings. He died in Strasbourg in 1967.

Jean François Marie Aicardi (1925-2015)

"If a man be gracious and courteous to strangers it shows he is a citizen of the world."
Francis Bacon (1625).

The most recent great neurologist to emerge from the Salpêtrière stable was a paediatrician.

The opening sentences of Jean Aicardi's obituaries say it all (almost):
"Jean Aicardi was arguably the greatest chid neurologist of the modern era."

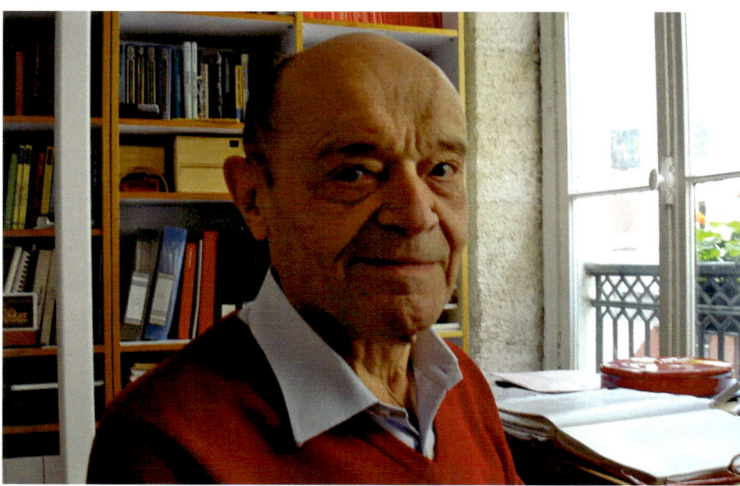

Jean François Marie Aicardi.

8. Perpetuating the Fame

John Stephenson, Professor of Paediatric Neurology, University of Glasgow, for the Child Neurology Society.

"*Jean Aicardi was a pioneering paediatric neurologist.*" Royal College of Physicians, *Inspiring Physicians* (Formerly Munk's Roll).

Add to those the entry in Wikipedia, and you'll appreciate the message:

"*He was known as one of the most distinguished and respected neuropediatricians of his time.*"

Jean Aicardi was born in the commune of Rambouillet some 27 miles southwest of Paris. He was the son of an engineer, one of nine children, two of whom died in infancy. He went to school in Versailles and studied medicine in Paris where he was an intern at the Salpêtrière. He graduated MD in 1955 with a dissertation on fits in the first year of life and in 1955-56 he held a research fellowship at Harvard and the Boston Children's Hospital.

In Paris he learnt neurology from Raymond Garcin, Guillain's son-in-law and one of the most distinguished of French neurologists, at the Salpêtrière and from Stéphane Thieffry, the first French paediatric neurologist at the *Hôpital des Enfants Malades*. He worked at the *Enfants Malades* and at the St. Vincent de Paul Hospital.

At the *Institut National de la Santé et de Recherche Médicale* (the National Institute for Health and Medical Research) (INSERM) he was master of research (1969-86) and director of research (1986-91). When he had to retire from INSERM in 1991 at the age of 65 he took up visiting professorships in Miami, in Sydney, and at the Institute of Child Health and Great Ormond Street Children's Hospital in London.

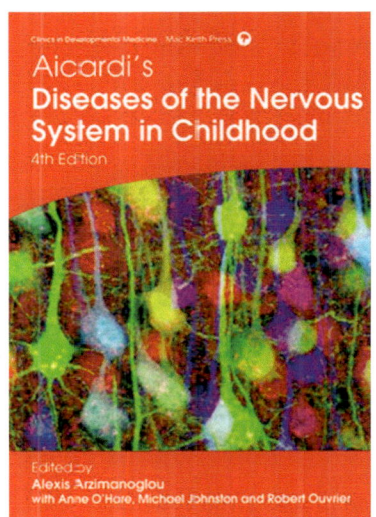

Jean Aicardi took paediatric neurology to the world both in person and with his books (he wrote in English). He gave his name to two rare diseases, Aicardi's syndrome (a severe form of epilepsy in infants with defects in the retina of the eye and agenesis of the corpus callosum, absence of the structure that connects the two sides of the brain); and with his colleague Françoise Goutières, Aicardi-Goutières syndrome, a rare form of brain disease in children. He was also prominent with others, in 'rediscovering' Rett syndrome, a brain disease of early childhood that affects only girls. He wrote over 250 papers on child neurology and he was the most peripatetic of child neurologists.

Rare diseases are common in paediatrics, by which I mean that when you add them all up together they're no longer so rare. So paediatricians have to be aware of the rarities. Very rare diseases have been called 'orphan' diseases, because it wasn't financially viable for the pharmaceutical companies to spend money looking for cures; they weren't going to sell many of them. But now they've been adopted. Almost each disease has a patient or parent group that speaks out loudly for their own disease and there are national provisions for the purpose. There are usually some doctors, even if it's only one or two in the country, who are experts on each individual disease. Paediatricians should know where to find them and if they don't the local parents' group will, or you just click onto the appropriate website. The problem is they have to be diagnosed in the first place, which may not be easy. The UK government published its UK Strategy for Rare Diseases in 2013 and in January this year (2021) there was a policy paper recommending that all four nations should produce an action plan before the end of the year "where possible". The European Organisation for Rare Diseases is called EURODIS; it could obviously be confused with a commercial outfit that gives pleasure to many children, although I see that's changed its name recently, perhaps for that reason.

Jean Aicardi was not only an excellent doctor, he was a good and humble man, he's also the only one in this book I ever met. That makes sense because he's the only one I have shared the planet with, at least as an adult. When he was in his late teens he experienced an utterly unspeakable tragedy when his brother Jacques was murdered in a nazi concentration camp. Was that what sparked off a lifetime of service to children with neurological problems? It's the eternal conflict, good against evil, smiles against tears, hope against despair, no better illustrated than in the history of the Salpêtrière Hospital. Rutger Bregman maintains that human beings are essentially good and kind and always have been since the beginning. I think he is correct on the whole but to my mind he has no adequate explanation for the terrible atrocities of history and of the present.

8. Perpetuating the Fame

The second invasion of the Salpêtrière

The Salpêtrière was invaded on 4 September 1792. Two hundred and twenty-six years and eight months later it was invaded again. On 1 May 2019 a group of protesters, *'gilets jaunes'* and others, entered the hospital; they gained access to the roof and were prevented from entering the intensive care unit only by the fortitude of the nursing staff. Luckily, on this occasion no hospital staff or patients came to any harm. There was rioting beyond the hospital, left wing marches are traditionally held on 'May Day'. The *Gilets Jaunes* were formed in November 2018 to protest against fuel tax rises but expanded into a general left wing movement. Protests are still being held in January 2021 but whether they are still *gilets jaunes* isn't clear. Holding your protest in a hospital is not, I believe, the very best of ideas.

Part 2

Beyond the Salpêtrière

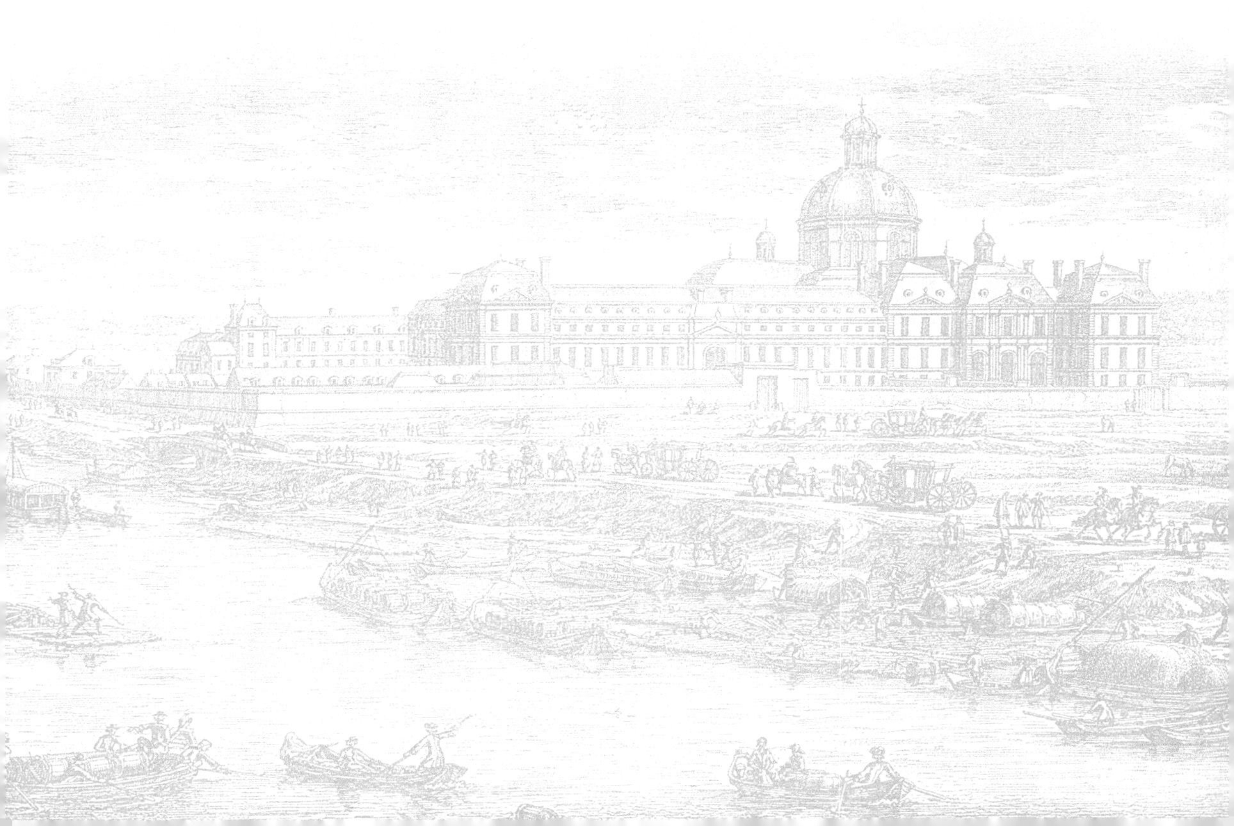

Chapter 9

Charcot's Contemporaries in Neurology

Brown-Séquard, Broca, Hughlings Jackson, Quincke, Gowers, Ramon y Cajal, Horsley, Alzheimer and Cushing

Charles Edouard Brown-Séquard (1817-1894)

Brown-Séquard is remembered for the spinal hemisection syndrome (Brown-Séquard syndrome). The arrangement of motor and sensory nerve tracts in the spinal cord is such that when the cord is split into two (right and left) halves, or almost halves, by injury or disease and one half is essentially destroyed a strange mixture of neurological findings occurs. There is paralysis on the same side of the body below the level of the damage but sensory ability is split according to the type of sensation. The ability to feel pain (or pinprick) is carried in different nerve tracts from the ability to feel touch or the position of a limb or part of a limb. Position sensation is tested by asking the patient to close their eyes and then moving a finger up or down and asking the patient to say up or down. In the spinal cord the nerve tracts that control movement of the right arm or leg are on the right side of the cord and those that control sensation to

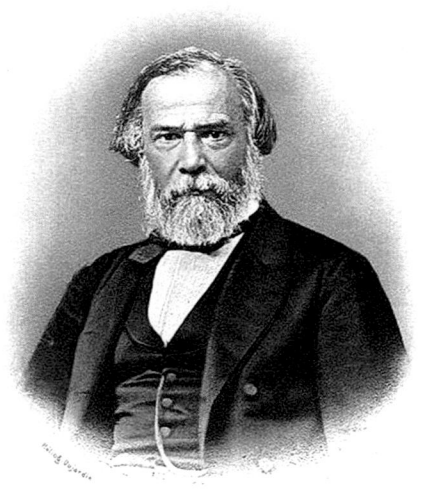

Charles Edouard Brown-Séquard.

touch or positon (that is the nerve tracts that carry the nerve impulses for these sensations to the brain) are also on the right. So damage to the right half of the cord will result in paralysis and in loss of touch and position sensation below the level of the damage on the right side of the body. But the nerve tracts that carry pain sensation to the brain cross over to the other side soon after entering the cord so sensation to pain is lost on the left side of the body below the level of the damage.

Brown-Séquard was born in Mauritius which had transferred from French to British control in 1817 but French culture was still strong and Brown-Séquard had both influences in his early life. His father was a sea captain who went down with his ship leaving his wife and child to fend for themselves. The boy, who had been born Charles Édouard Brown, then had his mother's name, Séquard, added. They moved to France and Brown-Séquard entered the Paris medical school, qualifying in 1846 but his mother died whilst he was a student. He worked on the function of the adrenal glands showing that they produced a substance that acted on other organs via the blood stream, in other words, a hormone. He therefore has a claim to recognition as one of the forerunners of endocrinology.

In 1854 he moved to the USA where he added to his reputation and taught at Harvard. On moving again, this time to England in 1859, he was involved in the founding of the National Hospital in Queen Square. He stayed there for another five years and later took up a chair at Harvard, but he moved again, back to France in 1878, to take over Claude Bernard's chair (see later) at the *Collège de France*. In 1868 he had collaborated with Charcot and Vulpian to found the *Archives de Physiologie*.

Brown-Séquard was clearly a brilliant man and perhaps he deserves to be remembered for more than his spinal hemisection syndrome, whilst acknowledging the intricate neurology of that syndrome. In his later life he was subjected to public derision for claiming to have rejuvenated himself by self-injecting with an extract of monkey testis.

Paul Pierre Broca (1824-1880)

Broca was born in the commune of Sainte-Foye-La-Grande in the Gironde department of southwest France. He trained in Paris, graduating MD in 1853 and became a surgical colleague of Charcot at the Salpêtrière. In 1847 and 1848 he joined first the Anatomical and then the Biological Society of Paris, increasing his scientific contacts, including Charcot. He developed an interest in anthropology and phrenology, developing theories that would now be dismissed as racist. He also became a supporter of Darwin and clashed with the Church. In his medical work he performed studies on bone and cartilage, cancer and aneurysms.

In 1861 at an anthropological meeting he showed the brain of a patient called Louis Leborgne who had recently died of gangrene and sepsis under his care. Leborgne had suffered from epilepsy from an early age and had suddenly stopped speaking at the age of 30, he could only say, "Tan, tan" and was thenceforth known as 'Tan'. Soon after stopping speaking, he gradually became paralysed down his right side. At autopsy Broca found lesions in the left frontal lobe. Thirty-six years previously a French physician called Jean-Baptiste Brouillard had claimed that patients with aphasia (loss of speech) always had damage to the front of the brain. Later in 1861 Broca had a second patient who was aphasic and had lesions almost identical to those of 'Tan'. In 1863 Broca presented a series of eight similar patients, some of whom had originally been patients of Charcot and whom Charcot had allowed him to include in his series. Broca had, for the first time, provided evidence of localisation of function within the brain whereas it had previously been thought that the brain functioned as a whole without its functions being localised to specific areas.

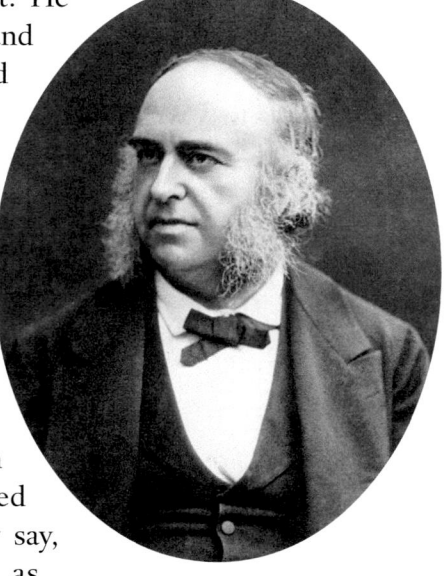

Paul Pierre Broca.

Broca's findings were disputed, particularly by Pierre Marie who in 1906 wrote a paper with the title, *The third convolution of the left frontal lobe does not play any special role in language function*. Amazingly, the preserved brains of Broca's two original patients were MRI-scanned in 2007 and their lesions were shown to extend beyond what has been regarded as Broca's area. Broca became celebrated as a scientist and he was later made a life senator in France. Seventy-two names are perpetuated on the Eiffel Tower; one of those names is Paul Broca.

John Hughlings Jackson (1835-1911)

John Hughlings Jackson has been described as the father of English neurology. He was born in Providence Green, Pontefract, Yorkshire on 4th of April 1835. His father, Samuel, was a brewer and a self-styled 'gentleman of the county', his mother was the daughter of the Collector of Excise for Halifax. He was the youngest of five children but his mother died not long after his first birthday and he was brought up by his father with whom he seems to have had a good relationship. He and his nearest brother were sent to a boarding school which he disliked intensely. At the age of 15 he was apprenticed to a GP in York and at 17 he enlisted at the small medical school in the same city (the new medical school of the Universities of Hull and York opened to students in 2003). After three years there he moved to London as a student at St. Bartholomew's Hospital where he came under the influence of Sir James Paget, a famous surgeon and pathologist, who became a longtime friend.

Hughlings Jackson took two qualifying exams: Licenciate of the Society of Apothecaries (LSA) and the dual Member of the Royal College of Surgeons and Licenciate of the Royal College of Physicians, (MRCS LRCP) having never been to a university. Later, in 1860, he submitted a thesis for the external MD degree of St. Andrews University. He was to become MRCP in 1860 and FRCP in 1866. After qualifying he returned to York to be Resident Medical Officer at the York Dispensary but in 1859 he was given an introduction to Dr. Jonathon Hutchinson who, although nine years older had had an almost identical career (born in Yorkshire, apprenticed to a GP in York, attended the York medical school, studied at St. Bartholomew's, protege of Sir James Paget, Resident Medical Officer at York General Hospital) and rented accommodation in Hutchinson's home in London.

That was the start of another lifelong friendship. Hutchison was to become Sir Jonathon Hutchinson, celebrated surgeon and medical polymath. For a while Hughlings Jackson earned a living as a

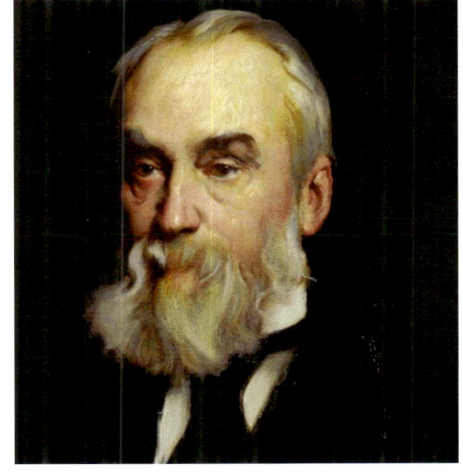

John Hughlings Jackson.

medical journalist in the general press and he met Brown-Séquard who put into his head the idea of becoming a neurologist. He joined the staff of the Metropolitan Free Hospital and then became a lecturer in pathology at the London Hospital. He was given a gold watch by the London Hospital for his work during England's cholera epidemic of 1862. John Snow had stopped the 1854 epidemic by removing the handle of the Broad Street pump, but that clearly didn't stop the next (and last) epidemic.

In 1859 a small hospital opened in London with just two consultants, Brown-Séquard and a doctor called J Z Ramskill. The new hospital was to become the nervous diseases hospital in Queen Square. When Brown-Séquard moved to the USA, Hughlings Jackson applied for the job but didn't get it, so when the new appointee resigned in 1867 Hughlings Jackson was appointed full physician to the National Hospital and stayed there for the rest of his career. He was one of the first physicians in the country to take to regular use of the ophthalmoscope after it was introduced by von Helmholtz in Berlin in 1851. He had been working as a clinical assistant at the Royal London Ophthalmic Hospital and the neurology of the eye became, and remained, one of his main interests. That hospital became Moorfields Eye Hospital. In 1874 he was appointed physician to the London Hospital and in 1878 he received the highly prestigious honour of being elected a Fellow of the Royal Society (FRS). He wrote a great deal but had a reputation for being a poor and at times almost incomprehensible writer.

Hughlings Jackson is chiefly remembered because of 'Jacksonian epilepsy'. This is the term used for fits that begin locally at some point such as the thumb and then spread up the limb until it crosses the midline when the patient becomes unconscious. The expression 'Jacksonian epilepsy' was promoted by Charcot who wrote that it was right that Jackson's name should be used in this context. Jackson pointed out that the involvement doesn't cease in the part where it starts as it moves on but collectively involves successive parts as it spreads. He became an expert on the subject of epilepsy as a whole. In showing that the fits originate in the motor cortex (outer layer) of the brain he enriched knowledge of the working of the brain and showed the way to surgical treatment for some forms of epilepsy. Like Charcot he insisted that a good doctor should have a thorough knowledge of pathology and that good medical practice and understanding began in the post-mortem room. He wrote a lot about aphasia addressing the minutiae of speech production and loss and emphasising that the problem was more complex than can be ascribed to a simple speech area whilst not denying the importance of that area. Jackson was a deep thinker about neurology, so deep as to be not readily understood by everyone. He is held in great respect by neurologists, Macdonald Critchley (1900-97), himself a very distinguished neurologist, ends his biography by quoting Wordsworth "Yet shall thy name conspicuous and sublime, stand in the spacious firmament of time, fixed as a star".

Heinrich Irenaeus Quincke (1842-1922)

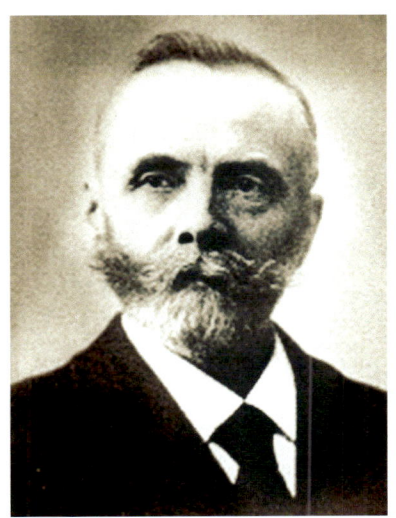

Heinrich Quincke.

Quincke is best remembered for introducing the technique of lumbar puncture in which a needle is inserted through the lower back to obtain cerebrospinal fluid for examination. Lumbar puncture was widely regarded as too dangerous until Quincke, in 1902, showed it to be feasible and safe and it became routine in the diagnosis or exclusion of meningitis, though there are still circumstances in which it is considered too dangerous.

Quincke was born in Frankfurt and studied in Heidelberg and Wurzburg before obtaining his doctorate in Berlin. He described the bounding pulse associated with malfunction (incompetence) of the aortic valve of the heart and also reported the condition of angioneurotic oedema an allergic condition to which there may be an inherited tendency in some cases. He was proposed for a Nobel Prize but was considered too old.

William Richard Gowers (1845-1915)

Macdonald Critchley (1900-97) a 20th century consultant at the Queen Square hospital and president of the World Federation of Neurology had a high opinion of, and respect for, his predecessors. He described John Hughlings Jackson as "the father of English neurology" and William Gowers as "probably the greatest clinical neurologist of all time".

Gowers' father was a bootmaker but he and three of William's siblings died when William was not yet eleven years old whereupon his mother went to live in Doncaster, leaving William in the care of relatives in Oxford where he attended Christ Church College School. On leaving school he was apprenticed to a GP in Essex where he was befriended by a minister of religion called Alfred Phipps. Phipps introduced him to Sir William Jenner, a famous and highly influential physician in London who became his mentor. Jenner was Professor of Medicine at University College, FRS and President of the Royal College of Physicians and not to be confused with Edward Jenner (1749-1823) of smallpox vaccination fame.

Gowers studied Medicine at UCL qualifying MRCS/LRCP in 1867, MB, BS in 1869 and graduating MD in 1870. He learned shorthand which helped him to take and keep notes, and the notes on his vast array of patients gave him the data for his books. At UCL he met John Russel Reynolds another early neurologist and future PRCP. Gowers was a registrar at Queen Square in 1870-72, becoming assistant physician and then full physician, and remaining there until he retired in 1910. He became Professor of Clinical Medicine at UCL in 1887 and was knighted in 1897.

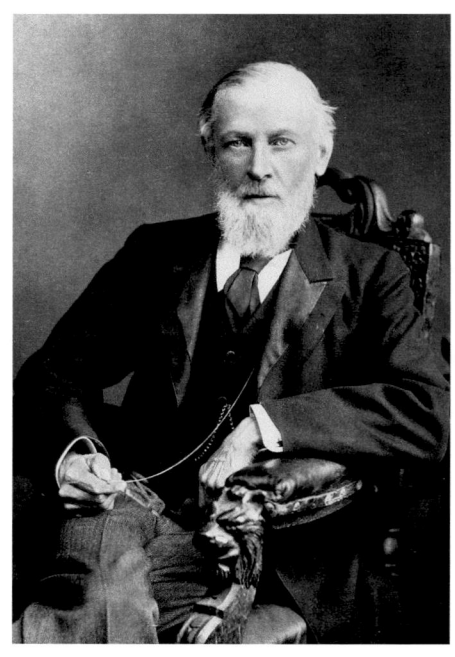

William Gowers.

Unlike Hughlings Jackson, he was a good writer and he expressed Jackson's precepts in a more comprehensible style. He was known as an excellent though dogmatic teacher. He invented an instrument for measuring haemoglobin concentration in blood (haemoglobinometer) and he produced the first patella hammer and was first to use the term 'knee jerk'. Boys with Duchenne type muscular dystrophy have a characteristic way of getting up from the floor, they get up into a crouching position then put their hands on their knees and 'climb up' their legs using their hands, Gowers was the first to describe this and it is known as Gowers' sign or manoeuvre. In 1886-8 he wrote his two volume *Manual of Diseases of the Nervous System* which is regarded as a, if not the, classic of neurological writing. Gowers wrote many influential books:

A Manual and Atlas of Medical Ophthalmoscopy (1879)
Pseudohypertrophic Muscular Paralysis (1879)
The Diagnosis of Diseases of the Spinal Cord (1880)
Epilepsy and other Chronic Convulsive Disorders, their Causes, Symptoms and Treatment (1881)
The Diagnosis of the Diseases of the Brain and of the Spinal Cord (1885)
Manual of Diseases of the Nervous System (2 volumes) (1886-8)
Syphilis and the Nervous System (1892)
The Dynamics of Life (1894)
Diagnosis of the Nature of Organic Brain Disease (1897)
Subjective Sensations of Sight and Sound, Abiotrophy and other lectures (1904)
The Borderland of Epilepsy: Faints, Vagal Attacks, Vertigo, Migraine, Sleep Symptoms and their treatment (1907)

Jackson and Gowers are remembered together as the giants of Queen Square and of British neurology. Jackson was a deep thinker, a modest and a gentle man; Gowers the supreme clinical neurologist, perhaps more outgoing and dogmatic.

Santiago Ramón y Cajal (1852-1934)

"His contribution to science was on a par with that of Vesalius."

Matthew Cobb, 2020.

Ramón y Cajal 'invented' the microscopic anatomy of the nervous system. He was born in Navarre in Spain and is said to have been a particularly rebellious boy. His father, who was a professor of anatomy, apprenticed him

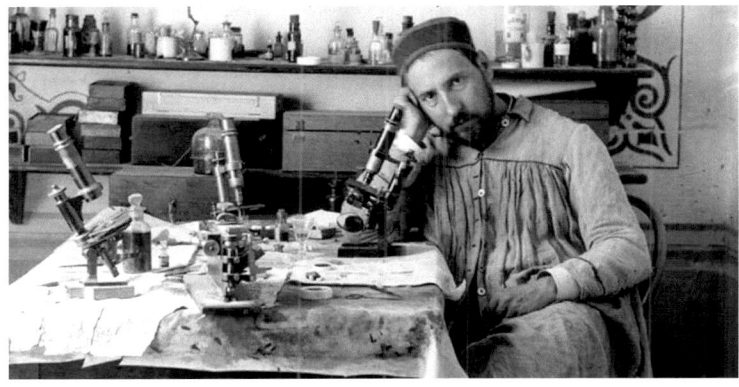

Santiago Ramón y Cajal.

as a teenager to first a shoemaker and then a barber in an attempt to quell his rebelliousness. He then attended Medical School in Zaragoza, graduating in 1873 and taking his MD in Madrid in 1877. He served in the Spanish army in Cuba in 1874-5. He held a series of anatomy professorships in Valencia, Barcelona and finally Madrid where he became director of the National Institute of Hygiene in 1899. He founded the Laboratory of Biological Investigations in 1922 which later became the Cajal Institute. At the end of the 19th century the predominant theory about the brain was the reticular theory which proposed that the brain was a continuous reticulum without individual cells. With his meticulous and painstaking use of the silver staining method for nerve cells discovered by the Italian scientist Golgi, Cajal showed that the nervous system is composed of separate cells with neurons that have axons that meet with other cells at synapses. The word synapse was introduced by Charles Sherrington in 1897. The Nobel Prize for Medicine in 1906 was won jointly by Cajal and Golgi, which caused a stir because Golgi was sticking to the reticular theory that Cajal had disproved using Golgi's stain. Cajal received many honours around the world and died in Madrid in 1934.

There have been two Spanish Nobel Laureates for Medicine, Cajal was the first and the second was Severo Ochoa in 1959 for studies on the synthesis of RNA and DNA.

Victor Alexander Haden Horsley (1857-1916)

Horsley was the father of English neurosurgery. He was born into an upper class family in Kensington. His father was a well-known artist and it is said that the names Victor and Alexander were chosen by Queen Victoria. He entered University College London in 1874 and the Hospital in 1875. He was a brilliant student, tipped for great things from early on and among his teachers were Gowers and Ringer of Ringer's solution fame. He qualified MRCS, LRCP in 1881 and was surgical registrar from 1882 to '84, taking the FRCS exam in 1883. He spent several years doing animal research and from 1884 to 1890 was professor-superintendent at the Brown Institution in London, a unit for animal research where he worked on localisation of brain function, thyroid research and following up Pasteur's work on a rabies vaccine (the Brown Institute fell into disuse and was closed in 1939, the building was destroyed by bombs in 1944).

It wasn't until 1890 that Horsley turned to full time clinical surgery, initially performing experimental thyroid transplant surgery. At first he was a general surgeon doing mainly thyroid surgery but he gradually moved to neurosurgery and was appointed to the National Hospital, Queen Square as well as University College Hospital. He became the first surgeon to operate successfully on a spinal tumour in 1887 on a patient of Gowers and extended his work to brain tumours. Babinski's neurosurgical colleague, De Martel, came from Paris to learn from him. He received a knighthood in 1902.

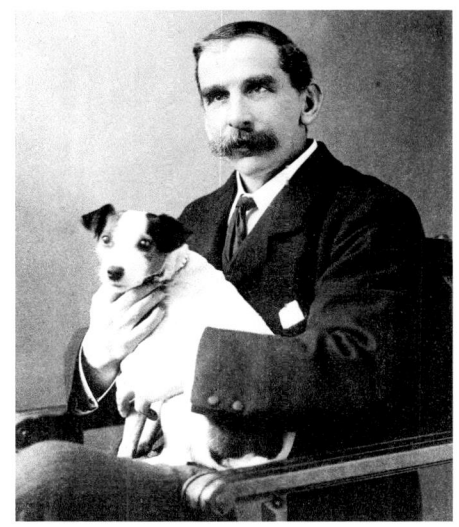

Victor Horsley.

Horsley did much more than his clinical work. He served on the General Medical Council for many years and took an interest in politics, both activities inviting criticism. He was an unsuccessful candidate for the Liberal Party on three occasions and a long-term campaigner against drink and smoking. During the First World War he rose to the rank of colonel in Egypt but in 1916 he became ill and died there aged 59. His death was attributed to overwork and sun-stroke.

Alois Alzheimer (1864-1915)

"When you forget I will remember for you
When you get lost I will find you."

From poem *I Will* by Michele DeSocio.

Alzheimer was born in a small town in Bavaria in 1864. He studied in Berlin, Tubingen and Wurzburg and graduated in medicine in 1887. The next year he took up a resident post at a hospital for the mentally ill and people with epilepsy in Frankfurt and stayed there for seven years. He met and formed a friendship and collaboration with Franz Nissl (1860-1919) after whom Nissl bodies, the site of protein synthesis in neurons, are named. They worked together on brain histopathology for seven years but in 1895 Nissl moved to Heidelberg to work

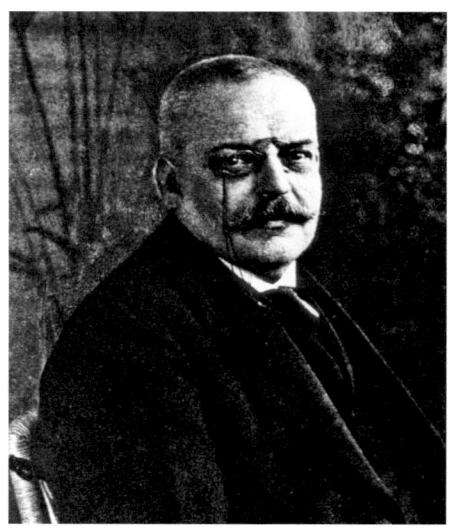
Alois Alzheimer (1864-1915).

with Emil Kraepelin (1856-1926), who is credited with being a founder of scientific psychiatry, and Alzheimer became director of the Asylum in Frankfurt. He had a patient there called Auguste Decker who had the symptoms of what used to be called presenile dementia.

Alzheimer then moved to Munich but arranged to have Decker's brain and records sent on to him when she died in 1906. On examination of the brain he found thinning of the cerebral cortex (outer layer) and on microscopy he found features called neurofibrillary tangles and amyloid plaques, features now known to be characteristic of the heart-breaking disease that is associated with his name. Alzheimer had moved to Heidelberg and Kraepelin in 1902 but moved again, to Munich, in 1903. In 1907 he had a second patient very much like Auguste Decker and with the same findings at autopsy. Kraepelin then called it Alzheimer's disease. Alzheimer accepted an associate professorship at the Psychiatric Institute in 1908 and a full professorship in Breslau in 1912 but by then he was ill and he died of heart disease in 1915 at the age of 51. It was a long time before the name Alzheimer's disease came into general use in the UK, when I was a young doctor in the early 1960s we still referred to it as presenile dementia but that was a rather nonspecific term. Alzheimer defined the disease, making the current intensive research possible.

Harvey Cushing (1869-1939)

Cushing is known, especially in America, as the father of neurosurgery. He was born on 8th April 1869 in Cleveland, Ohio, the youngest of ten children. The first of the family in America, Matthew Cushing, had sailed into Boston from Gravesend in 1638. Harvey's father, grandfather and great grandfather had all been GPs. He received his early education in Cleveland and went on to Yale from 1887 to 1891 before entering Harvard Medical School in Boston in September 1891. Charcot, Gowers and Cushing were all fine draughtsmen but Cushing in later life complained of having 'lost the touch'.

Cushing graduated MD *cum laude* in June 1895 and began his first post at the Massachusetts General Hospital. In October of that year he visited the Johns Hopkins Hospital in Baltimore and met both Osler and Halsted, probably the most highly regarded physician and surgeon in the country at that time, or shortly after. The Johns Hopkins Hospital had opened in 1889 and when, in 1910, Abraham Flexner produced his Flexner Report on American medical schools he castigated most of them but pointed to the Johns Hopkins school, opened in 1893, as the example to be followed by all the rest. Halsted's pupils went on to fill many of the most prestigious posts in surgery around the USA. Cushing wrote to Halsted asking for a job but was told that the jobs at Johns Hopkins were all taken and he would be better off spending some time in Europe. He intended to go to Vienna but circumstances at Johns Hopkins changed and Halsted offered him a place in 1896. Although he had great respect for Halsted he didn't take to him as he did to Osler. He lived next door to Osler and they became friends, Cushing was later to write a much praised two volume *Life of Osler* that he described as a labour of love.

Osler had a very extensive library and he would give a latch key to his house to the senior residents he particularly favoured so that they had access to the library, Cushing became one of Osler's 'latch key men'. Incidentally Cushing in his Osler biography refers to a meeting in Folkestone in 1881, associated with the London international medical conference of that year, which was attended by Pasteur, Lister, Virchow, Huxley, Paget, Hughlings Jackson, Charcot and Koch – a more distinguished gathering of medics it would be difficult to imagine.

Halsted saw great promise in Cushing and he became Halsted's resident in 1897, a post he kept for four years, much of that time he had to stand on his own two feet. Halsted was experimenting with local anaesthesia and, not realising the potential for addiction injected himself repeatedly with cocaine and became addicted, like Marie Curie and her radium he didn't anticipate the danger. His

Harvey Cushing.

health deteriorated and he was frequently away from work. Luckily Cushing was a born surgeon and although called upon to perform surgery beyond what ought to have been expected of him, he thrived. He also occasionally gave general anaesthetics and developed a routine of frequent monitoring of pulse and respiratory rates during anaesthesia. He called the recordings ether charts and later, after a visit to Italy, he added blood pressure monitoring having obtained an early mercury sphygmomanometer in Pavia (the mercury sphygmomanometer was invented by Scipione Riva-Rocci a physician, pathologist and paediatrician at the University of Padua not long before Cushing's visit and Cushing was among the first to introduce it into the United States).

Soon after taking up his post Cushing developed appendicitis. At that time appendicectomy (my computer wants me to write appendectomy but I'm not going to) was regarded as a dangerous procedure and Halsted was reluctant to operate but Cushing persuaded him to do so. Cushing was first in the field in many ways, when he arrived in Baltimore he brought with him from Boston an X-ray machine and for a while he was the only person at Johns Hopkins to take and interpret X-rays. Roentgen had announced his discovery of X-rays in 1895. Yet another novelty popularised in the USA by Cushing was the use of Ringer's solution for intravenous infusion. Ringer had developed the electrolyte solution while working on isolated frogs heart preparations at University College in London in the early 1880s showing that calcium and potassium were essential components of the mixture.

In 1900-01 Cushing spent 14 months in Europe visiting, most importantly, Charles Sherrington the physiologist in Liverpool and Theodor Kocher, the surgeon, in Berne. He was impressed by Sherrington and did animal work in his laboratory on the localisation of function in the cerebral cortex. He didn't feel that he gained much from Kocher but worked on brain physiology in the laboratory of Hugo Kronecker, an elderly but distinguished physiologist. He watched Horsley operate in London but considered him a slapdash surgeon (his feelings about Horsley improved later).

Back at Johns Hopkins, Halsted had a small space for teaching surgery to students on animals (that no longer happens). In 1903 Cushing appealed for funds to build a new unit and the Hunterian Laboratory for Experimental Medicine opened in 1905. As well as teaching surgery the new unit provided a veterinary service to the local population (as did the Brown Institute in London) and further room for Cushing's animal research. It was here that he elucidated the workings of the pituitary gland. Halsted started handing over patients with neurological problems to Cushing and the results of head and spine operations were at first dismal but they gradually improved. In 1910 Cushing was joined in the Hunterian Laboratory by Walter Dandy who was himself to become a distinguished neurosurgeon but then was Cushing's resident. They were incompatible and became lifelong rivals, they were two alpha males in the same territory. Cushing was an autocrat who didn't tolerate opposition and Dandy was annoyed when Cushing told him, late in the day, that he was not going to take him with him to Harvard when he left in 1912 to take up the chair of surgery at Harvard University and the Peter Bent Brigham Hospital in Boston. Around this time he saw a patient with a previously unrecognised set of signs and symptoms, but with his knowledge of pituitary composition and function he suggested that the problem was a certain type of tumour of the pituitary gland, a basophil adenoma, that was secreting too much ACTH (adreno-cortico-trophic hormone). As the name implies that hormone stimulates the cortex of the adrenal gland above the kidney to produce more cortisone. Many years later (1932) he published all the accumulated evidence showing that his suggestion was correct.

At Harvard Cushing concentrated on neurosurgery and, as Halsted had done in general surgery, trained many assistants who became professors or chiefs of neurosurgery at universities and hospitals around the USA. In the First World War he led a Harvard unit in France and in the summer of 1917 he was working with the British army in a medical field station near Passchendaele. On the 26 of August he received a letter from Grace Osler the wife of William Osler, then the most famous physician in the English speaking world (I typed in the word 'arguably' and then deleted it), saying that their son Revere, a lieutenant in the British army, was serving in the same area and remarking how awful it would be if he were seriously injured and became a patient of Cushing, though lucky in his surgeon (Cushing was a close and longstanding friend of the Oslers). Late on the 29th he, now Major Cushing, got a message that Lieutenant Osler was seriously injured and in a casualty clearing station a few miles away. Cushing was driven to the station and by midnight was operating together with three other of America's most prominent surgeons, but Revere died the next morning. He was 21. They wrapped him in a Union Jack and buried him in "a soggy Flanders field, beside a little oak grove" (*"If I should die, think only this of me… some corner of a foreign field"*).

Revere Osler had been born in America and schooled in England, he was attended by American surgeons and when he died was wrapped in a Union Jack. The shell that struck Revere's trench killed two Oslers because on the 29 of December 1919 Sir William Osler died in Oxford of pneumonia, but almost certainly the underlying cause was intense and persisting grief. In his diary he had written that he'd had a wonderful life and almost everything he had hoped for had happened; he had been a happy man, but then he wrote, "Call no man happy until he is dead." Osler had always delighted in children and loved to play with them, he was 46 when his only son was born. Revere was given that name because he was descended on his mother's side from an American hero. He was the great, great grandson of Paul Revere, who is honoured in American history for his night time ride (later mythologised by Longfellow) to warn the American forces of the arrival of the British at the start of the War of Independence in 1775. And yet here was Paul Revere's great, great grandson, a lieutenant in the British army, being buried wrapped in a Union Jack.

The senior Osler was born to Cornish missionary parents on the Canadian forest frontier and made his name at the new Johns Hopkins Hospital in Baltimore before becoming Regius Professor of Medicine in the University of Oxford in his maturity. He was a general physician treating patients of all ages but he was instrumental in the development of paediatrics in America, a founder member and third president of the American Pediatric Society (Americans don't like diphthongs). I have a strong suspicion that had he been born 50 or more years later he might well have been a paediatrician. That's why I personally hold him in such regard (Paediatrics in the USA didn't really get going until the 20th century and in England it was later than in the USA).

Considering his personality, it is perhaps not surprising that whilst in the army Cushing nearly got himself court-martialled for disregarding regulations. In 1918 he developed what is now recognised as Guillain-Barré syndrome from which he never recovered completely. Between 1920 and 1924, he devoted himself to writing his *Life of Sir William Osler* for which he was awarded the Pulitzer Prize, although one cynic described it as simply a copy and paste version of Osler's many outgoing and incoming letters, Cushing wouldn't have been familiar with the expression 'copy and paste'. In 1933 he returned to his *Alma Mater* Yale, as professor of neurology. He was embraced by academia in his final years, just as Einstein was in Princeton some years later. He was nominated for a Nobel Prize many times. He died of a heart attack in New Haven, Connecticut in 1939.

Cushing was clearly a supremely talented and driven man who could accept no less than perfection in himself or others, a trait for which he paid in human relationships. He would drive nurses to tears and his junior staff to despair with his scorn and sarcasm but he was undoubtedly a very great surgeon, pathologist and physiologist. An historian, the author of a Cushing biography, speaking to an audience that included Cushing's family at the dedication of his library and museum to Yale, said in true American style, "The question is whether or not he was an egotistical, hard driving, selfish, mean son-of-a-bitch." Which I think translates on the right-hand side of the pond into a sexually restricted version of p in the a. The question *is* how much does the world gain from a son-of-a-bitch (or p in the a) genius? Since, by definition, genius is rare I reckon we can put up with a few, the balance is positive, so long as they don't wander onto our patch, of course.

"He may be a son of a bitch but he's our son of a bitch."

President Franklin D Roosevelt, about Samoza the notorious dictator of Nicaragua.

Chapter 10

Charcot's Contemporaries in Biological Science

Claude Bernard (1813-1878)

"Physiology is the stepchild of medicine."

Martin H Fischer (1879-1962).

"Until one has loved an animal a part of one's soul remains unawakened."

Anatole France (1844-1924).

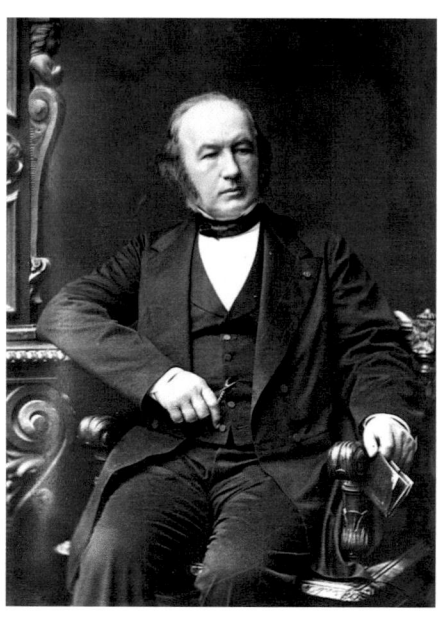

Claude Bernard.

Claude Bernard was possibly the most famous of all physiologists although today he would be condemned (I believe quite rightly) as a cruel vivisectionist.

He was born in the small town of Saint-Julien en Beaujolais in the Rhône department into a wine-making family. At the age of 19 he took a job as assistant to a local pharmacist but after 19 months he was sacked after making a mistake with a prescription. He then entered on a career in vaudeville and the theatre but on seeking advice from a professor of literature at the Sorbonne he was steered towards medicine on the grounds that he already had experience in the pharmacy. There have been quite a few medics who have made it on the stage or in the theatre, probably the most noted being Jonathan Miller. Must be something in the joint evolutionary heritage, though I'm very definitely in the non-vaudevillian branch of the family.

Bernard enrolled at the Paris medical school in 1834 and graduated MD in 1843 with a thesis on the role of gastric juice in nutrition. He worked at the Charité hospital in Paris and then moved to the Hôtel-Dieu and the Salpêtrière. At the Hôtel-Dieu he met the distinguished physiologist and anatomist, Magendie and worked as his assistant from 1841 to 1844 when he failed the *agrégation* exam and came into dispute with Magendie, but peace between the pair was restored by Professor Rayer, the mentor of Charcot, and Bernard subsequently followed Magendie in his professorial chair at the Collège de France. Bernard was a member of the influential Biological Society of Paris where he would meet Charcot and other clinicians. He was a vivisectionist before the introduction of anaesthesia, a practice which would not now be tolerated, and he encountered much opposition. His wife and daughters joined the campaigns against vivisection.

Bernard made many important discoveries in physiology. He showed that the liver stored glycogen as a sugar reserve and demonstrated the role of bile in protein digestion. He clarified the digestive function of the pancreas and showed the role of the red cells and haemoglobin in carrying oxygen around the body. He worked on the physiology of the heart, showing that the vagus nerve controlled the heart beat frequency and he demonstrated the actions of the sympathetic nervous system in constricting and dilating the blood vessels. He is most famous for showing in his experiments between 1851 and 1878 the preservation of the inner body environment, what he called the *milieu intérieur,* the maintenance of the temperature and chemistry of the body tissues within certain limits.

He wrote his best known book *Introduction to the study of experimental medicine* in 1865. Louis Pasteur had attended his lectures and they became great mutual admirers but they later disagreed about the philosophy of science, induction versus deduction, whether it is better to look for facts to build a theory or to develop a theory and then seek experimental proof or falsification. Deduction is the favourite, or at least it was when I was most active. The Emperor Napoleon III befriended them both and aided their work. Bernard died in 1878 and was given a state funeral, the first scientist to be awarded that honour.

It's now impossible to 'undiscover' his contributions to physiology. Medicine would be a broken science if we tried to. There have been many cruel experiments in the history of medicine; we can only hope to make kind use of the knowledge so gained, but I fully accept the proposition that we are all creatures of our own times, apart from those exceptional people who change the thinking of their times, like Pinel and Charcot, but even they remained creatures of their own times in many ways.

Louis Pasteur (1822-1895)

"In the field of observation, chance favours only the prepared mind."

Pasteur, 1845.

The name of Pasteur is known universally because of the process of Pasteurisation. Pasteur was born in 1822 in Dole in the Jura department of eastern France into a family of limited means, his father was a tanner. He showed no signs of exceptional ability at school but did have a flair for drawing and painting. He studied philosophy in Besancon and science in Dijon and in 1843 at the second time of asking got into the *École Normale Supérieure* (ENS), the highly prestigious graduate school in Paris. He taught physics at the College of Tournon in the Ardeche but was soon back at the ENS doing research into crystallography. In 1848 he moved to Strasbourg as professor of chemistry and there he met his wife, Marie Laurent, the daughter of the university's rector. They went on to have five children, three of whom died of typhoid in childhood.

Back at the ENS between 1857 and 1867 he was director of scientific studies, but with his dictatorial attitude he caused much dissention and alienated many students. His next move was to the Sorbonne where he was professor of organic chemistry from 1867 until he founded the Pasteur Institute in 1887. At the ENS and in Strasbourg he had performed ground breaking work on molecular asymmetry. Working with solutions of tartaric acid, he discovered the phenomenon of molecular isomerism, in which molecules of the same substance rotate light in different directions, some to the left (levorotatory) and some to the right (dextrorotatory).

He began studies on the fermentation of wine in 1856 showing the importance of yeast in the process and that micro-organisms were responsible for beer, wine and milk going sour. He introduced the process of moderate heating to prevent it happening (pasteurisation). He later went on to study the diseases of silkworms which were ruining the silk industry. Beware of the things that 'everybody knows', in the mid-19th century everybody knew that living organisms could arise by spontaneous generation, after all, Aristotle had taught us so. Pasteur demolished the theory with his famous experiments with broth in swan necked flasks, the broth didn't 'go off' if the bend in the swan neck protected it but did so if 'dust' was allowed to enter, thus it was the 'dust' not the air itself that contained microbes. In order to disprove spontaneous generation though, you would have to show the real method of generation, which I don't think Pasteur did.

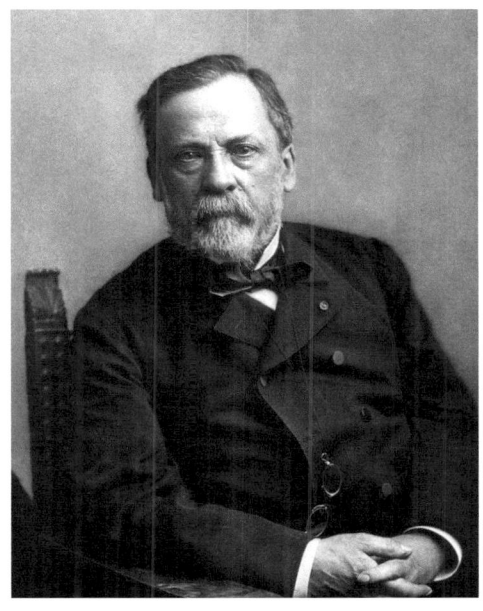

Louis Pasteur.

Pasteur then worked on chicken cholera and on anthrax in sheep, goats and cows producing prototype vaccines and attracting criticism from none other than the great Robert Koch, the discoverer of the tubercle bacillus, the cause of tuberculosis. In the 1880s a physician colleague of Pasteur, Émile Roux developed a vaccine against rabies, which was a much feared disease at that time. Pasteur tested it on a boy who had been attacked by a rabid dog. The boy did not develop rabies but it has since been said that he only had a small risk of getting it anyway. Pasteur had put himself on the wrong side of the law by treating the boy when he was not medically qualified. The rabies vaccine ran into much controversy but Charcot gave it strong support at the Academy of Medicine though Charcot himself never got into 'germ theory'. Pasteur was present at the dinner at Charcot's home when Charcot suffered his first significant attack of cardiac pain. In 1886 Sir Victor Horsley was secretary to a government commission to look into the rabies vaccine and subsequently campaigned in favour of its use throughout the United Kingdom.

Pasteur had a stroke with left hemiparesis (paralysis of the left side of the body) in 1868 but recovered. He died in 1895 after another stroke and was given a state funeral. He was buried in Notre-Dame Cathedral but his remains were later moved to the Pasteur Institute.

Pasteur's lab books were kept in secret (at his request) by the family for many years until in 1964 his grandson gave them to the *Bibliothèque National de France*. In 1995 on the 100th anniversary of Pasteur's death they were published, together with the accusation that he had falsified some of the entries. In the storm that followed, the unattractive side of his character came out.

Charles Scott Sherrington (1857-1952)

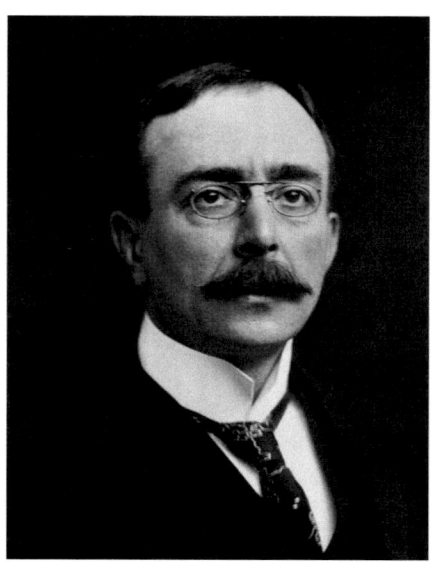

Charles Sherrington.

Sherrington was one of the greatest neurophysiologists of the early 20th century. He was born on 27 November 1857 but his origins present as an intriguing, hilarious, kaleidoscopic gallimaufry (or gallimaufric kaleidoscope if you prefer) of different theories. He was born in Islington, London, or perhaps India, or even Ipswich (no not Ipswich). His mother was Anne Sherrington or perhaps Brookes (her pre-marital name was Thurtell and it doesn't seem clear where the Brookes came from). His father was not James Norton Sherrington who was not a country doctor as had been suggested, but an ironmonger in Islington who died in 1848. He was the son of Caleb Rose who was a well-known surgeon in Ipswich or a classical scholar, archaeologist and art lover, or all three or four of the above. The name Caleb seems to introduce a kind of 'call me Ishmael'-ish flavour into this already Shakespearean Comedy-like miscellany of confusions. The family (Caleb, Anne, Charles and two brothers) moved from Islington to Ipswich in 1860. Caleb Rose married Anne in 1880 when his first wife died and they seemed to find stability and happiness in Ipswich.

After attending Ipswich School, Charles, apparently none the worse for all that, became a medical student in 1876 at Cambridge University, linked for clinical teaching and experience to St. Thomas's Hospital in London. In 1879 he studied physiology at Cambridge entering Gonville and Caius College. He attended a conference in London in 1881 and became firmly hooked on neurophysiology. He subsequently became a demonstrator in anatomy at Cambridge and then in histology at St. Thomas's.

During 1884-85 Sherrington studied in Strasbourg under Friedrich Goltz who had taken up the chair of physiology there two years previously. Goltz was a neurophysiologist who believed that the brain acted as a whole without localisation of function (the reticular theory). Sherrington, who was to become one of the people who scotched that idea, passed his medical qualifying exams in 1884 and obtained a first class honours degree in Natural Sciences, with distinction, at Cambridge the next year. He was an athlete and represented his college at rowing and played rugby for St. Thomas's and football for Ipswich Town.

In 1891 he followed Victor Horsley as professor and superintendent at the Brown Institute for Advanced Physiology and Pathology Research in London before taking up the chair of physiology in Liverpool where he supervised Cushing for eight months. He became the Waynfleet professor of Physiology in Oxford in 1913, his life's work was on the physiology of the nervous system in animals. He introduced the word 'synapse' into the scientific vocabulary and showed that the actions of the nervous system were integrated; a reflex arc was not just a simple arc because stimulation (contraction) of one muscle was always accompanied by relaxation of the corresponding opposing muscles. His books included *The Integrated Action of the Nervous System* (1906) and *Mammalian physiology: a course of practical exercises* (1919) the latter of which is regarded as a classic.

During the First World War Sherrington was chairman of the Industrial Fatigue Board and worked long hours at a shell factory in Birmingham. He was knighted in 1922 and together with Edgar Adrian (Lord Adrian) he was awarded the Nobel Prize in 1932. They both achieved OM (Order of Merit) and PRS (President of the Royal Society). Having reached an age of philosophical reflection in wartime in 1940 he published *Man on his Nature*, after he had retired in 1936 and returned to Ipswich. He died suddenly of heart disease in a nursing home in Eastbourne in 1952 aged 94. There is a commemorative stained-glass window in the dining hall of Gonville and Caius College.

Part 3

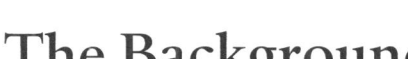

The Background

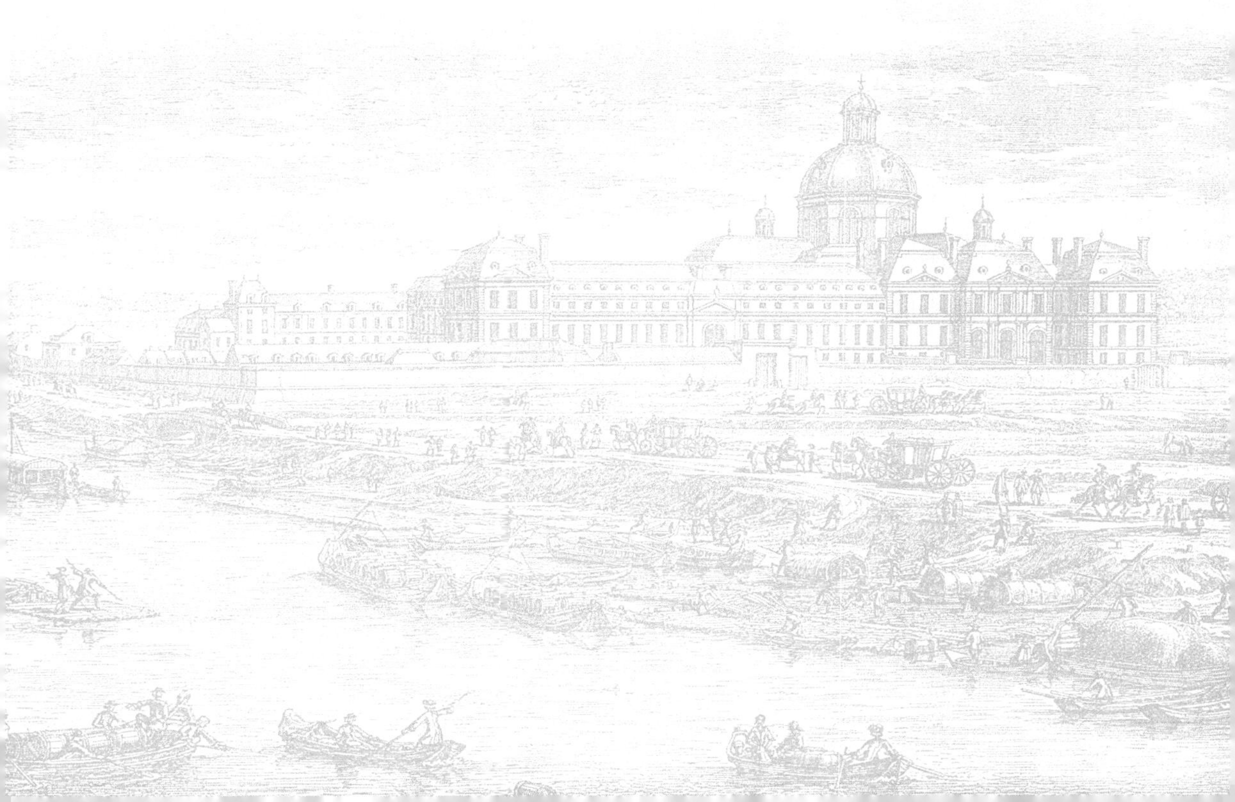

France in the Time of Charcot

The Contemporary Scene: Governance 1814-1914

France 1814-1914

It is not within the scope of this book to discuss the reign of Napoleon Bonaparte. To provide background to the period of the main development of the hospital I shall briefly summarise the situation in the country, but particularly in Paris, from just before to just after the life of Charcot. Table 1 is a guide to the governance of the country from the revolution to the present.

Table 1 – French Governance since the 1st Republic

1792-1804

- 1st Republic
- During the Revolution: The National Convention from 20th September 1792 to 3rd November 1795. The Directory from 3rd November 1795 to 9th November 1799
- Under Napoleon: Napoleon Bonaparte as 1st Consul from 22nd September 1799 to 18th May 1804

1804-1814

- 1st Empire
- Emperor Napoleon the first
- 1814 (disputed)
- For 15 days, June-July. Emperor Napoleon II, Son of Napoleon I

1814-1824 (interrupted by Napoleon's 100 days in 1815)

- Bourbon Restoration
- King Louis XVIII

1824-1830
- King Charles X
- 1830 2nd Revolution

1830-1848
- House of Orleans
- King Louis Philippe. 'July Monarchy'

1848-1851
- Second Republic
- President Louis Napoleon Bonaparte

BECAME:

1852-1870
- Second Empire
- Emperor Napoleon III

1870-1940
- Third Republic

1940-1944
- French State. Occupied France. (Vichy Government)

1944-1946
- Provisional Government of the French Republic
- De Gaulle

1946-1958
- Fourth Republic

1958-present
- Fifth Republic

Chapter 11

The Bourbon Restoration (1814-1830)

Louis XVIII

By the end of 1813 many of the French had had enough of their Emperor's endless wars and the shambles in Russia with the retreat from Moscow, together with increasing poverty, meant that he had lost much of his support. The allied armies against Napoleon were closing in on Paris and by the end of March 1814 they entered the city and he was forced to abdicate on 6th April and exiled to the Mediterranean island of Elba, a 'stone's throw' from his home island of Corsica. The allies then had the headache of deciding to whom they would give the job of ruling France and, for lack of a better option, they decided to bring back the Bourbons in the shape of the Count of Provence, who was the natural heir to the throne and younger brother of the King the French had decapitated 21 years previously.

The son of Louis XVI was a young child when his father was executed. He was proclaimed Louis XVII by royalists but died in prison, still a child. The new man on the throne was therefore Louis XVIII. When Napoleon skipped out of Elba in March 1815 for his 100 days of

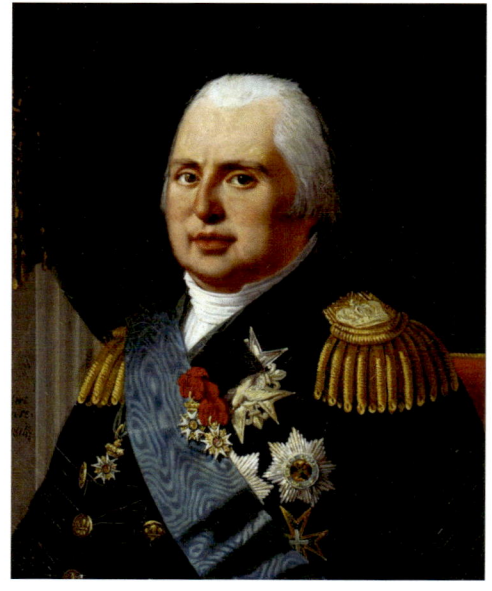

King Louis XVIII.

11. The Bourbon Restoration (1814-1830)

freedom, Louis XVIII fled the country until Napoleon was finally crushed at Waterloo on 18th June, forced to abdicate for the second time and sent to his well-guarded seclusion on the island of St. Helena, some 47 square miles of British land in the South Atlantic, around 1,200 miles off the coast of southwest Africa, from which even he could not think of escaping and where he died on 5th May 1821. He was entombed at *Les Invalides* in Paris in 1840.

Even considerably more than a century after 'old Boney' died, English children were still threatened with 'the bogey man will get you'. I can remember it being said, laughingly, when I was very young and having it explained when I was older that 'old boney' and the 'bogey man' both referred to Bonaparte. I remember too that in a drawer at home there was a small bronze likeness of Napoleon that I was allowed to play with and did at times. I think the English had a certain amount of respect for their old enemy long after he was gone because similar models of Boney were fairly common.

In 1814 the new King (Louis XVIII) had signed a Constitutional Charter which left him very much still the number one honcho. In it, the person of the King was deemed 'sacred and inviolable' and the sole holder of 'executive power'. It did, however, include provision for personal liberty, equality before the law, a bicameral parliament and the right of that parliament to control taxation. Louis XVIII had a troubled reign dealing with factions from extreme monarchist (the ultras) to extreme left (the Bonapartists) and it was one of the latter who assassinated the Duc De Barry, his nephew and the son of his successor Charles X, at the Paris Opera in February 1820.

After Napoleon's final downfall in 1815 those who had supported him during the '100 days' were hounded; some prosecuted and others lynched. Napoleon's Marshal Ney was executed in what became known as the second White Terror; the first was during the revolution. The second was mainly in the south of France, in Provence and Languedoc. Louis died in September 1824 suffering from obesity, gout and gangrene of the legs.

Charles X

Louis XVIII's brother was even less inclined towards constitutional monarchy and was to precipitate the second revolution in 1830.

Charles X didn't stand for much 'nonsense' about his lack of divine rights. He was a very strong supporter of the Church, bringing in severe punishment for sacrilege, promoting Church affairs and he even trying to introduce the practice

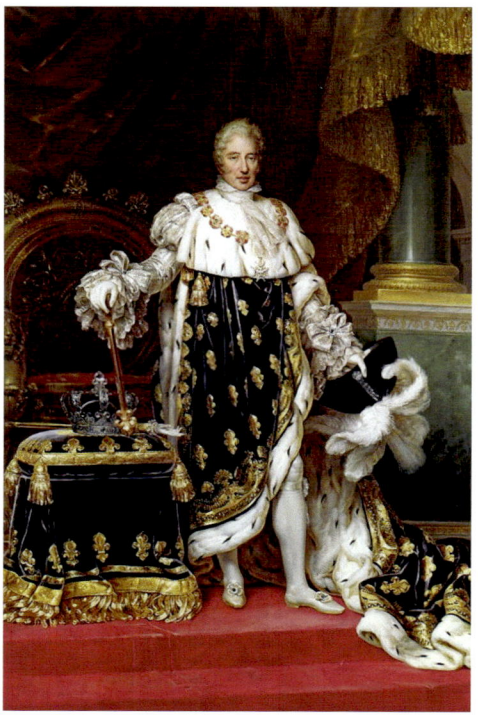

Charles X.

of 'the Royal Touch' whereby the touch of the King would cure scrofula (tuberculosis of the lymph glands in the neck). A double blind trial would have been fairly easy to do, all you'd need would be a doppelganger placebo King, and you wouldn't have needed many participants, but who needs that when you're carrying out the work of the deity?

His regime became increasingly authoritarian. He dissolved the lower chamber of parliament in 1830 and barricades appeared again in the streets of Paris. Troops, subjected to stone-throwing, fired without orders on the crowd and in the subsequent riot 850 people, crowd and military, were killed and it became the second French Revolution. This is the revolt pictured

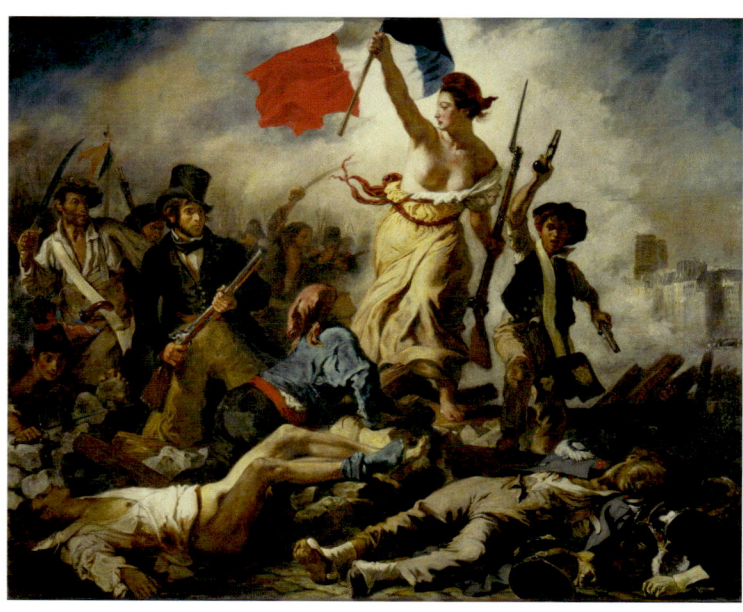

Liberty leading the People.

11. The Bourbon Restoration (1814-1830)

in the famous Delacroix painting of *Liberty leading the People* often taken as representing the 1789 revolution. Charles X abdicated and handed the throne to the Duc d'Orléans, a more distant member of the Bourbon family.

King Louis Philippe

He reigned from 1830 to 1848 as King Louis Philippe and his reign is known as the July monarchy in the House of Orléans of which he was the only occupant. It too was to end in revolution. Initially he was a popular monarch having been educated when young in Enlightenment values, proving much more lenient than his predecessors and ruling under a constitution that put power much more in the hands of parliament. He had proved himself a brave, patriotic and effective military commander in the Revolutionary Wars of the early 1790s and before taking the throne he had spent 21 years in exile in Switzerland, England and the USA, working for a living from time to time as a schoolteacher. He survived an assassination attempt in 1835 but by 1848 political and economic strife led to his downfall and the start of the Second Republic.

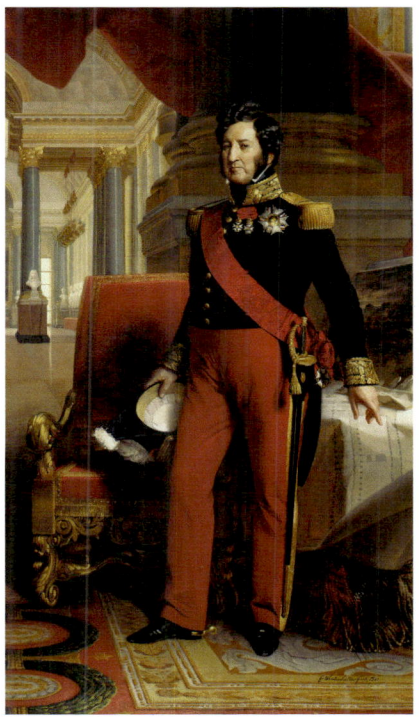

Louis Philippe.

Second Republic

President Louis Napoleon

In the election that followed the abdication of Louis Philippe, Bonaparte's nephew, Louis Napoleon won a large majority and became president of the Second Republic but that didn't last long because when he was barred by the constitution from running for a second term as president he staged a coup d'etat in 1852, and was proclaimed Emperor Napoleon III (Bonaparte's son had been declared Napoleon II by his supporters, briefly, after his father's final defeat, but he never ruled).

Second Empire

Emperor Napoleon III

Many people accepted what was on the whole a fairly liberal regime especially after French patriotism was boosted by victory in the Crimean war of 1853-56 to which the French contributed far more manpower than the British. The Emperor increased public spending as well as attracting private investment and his prefect of the Seine, Baron Haussmann, between 1852 and 1870 supervised the rebuilding of the city centre, providing wide boulevards, parks, a new sewage system and removal of the slums. The wide avenues made it more difficult to erect barricades and for that reason some complained that the works had a military purpose, to aid the suppression of rebellion. Others were simply saddened at the disappearance of their old haunts or tired of the endless building work. It all built up into a considerable opposition to Haussmann and after being defended by the Emperor initially, he was sacked in 1870, although the work went on after that for more than 50 years.

In 1870 the Emperor made his big mistake. He decided to take on the much superior Prussian army. As the last French monarch to lead his army in the field he was captured during the battle of Sedan. The Prussians besieged Paris causing much stress to the people of the city including the nursing sister Marguerite Bottard who was caught up in the fighting on one of her rare missions of mercy outside the grounds of the Salpêtrière. A humiliating peace deal was arranged in which France lost Alsace and Lorraine and the Prussian army marched triumphantly through the streets of Paris. The Third Republic was proclaimed and lasted from 1871 to 1940. The first part of the Third Republic (up to 1914) was looked upon in retrospect, after the horrors of 1914-18, as the Good Times, *La Belle Époque*. Before the good times, however, Paris had to suffer one more terrible, if brief, calamity.

Charles-Louis Napoleon.

Chapter 12

The Paris Commune of 1871

In 1871 after the humiliation of the Franco-Prussian war, and the siege that caused widespread near or actual starvation, Paris was in a state of agitated anxiety, a tinderbox ready to explode with political right-left divisions. The spark came on the Butte (hill or mound) of Montmartre with a dispute about cannons. Like the Duke of York's 10,000 men the 200 cannons had been dragged to the top of the hill by the people (*the Communards*) but the government claimed ownership and wanted to drag them down again. In the scuffle that followed two government generals were captured and shot and that caused an almighty conflagration. The Communards set up their own government in opposition to the one led by Adolphe Thiers that had negotiated the much resented settlement with the Prussians. The week of the 21st to the 28th of May 1871 will never be forgotten in France and has forever after been known as 'the Bloody Week'. Atrocity was followed by counter atrocity with mass executions on both sides. Perhaps the most egregious was at the Père-Lachaise cemetery where, after a gunfight, the surviving 147 Communards were lined up against a wall and shot, they were then buried in

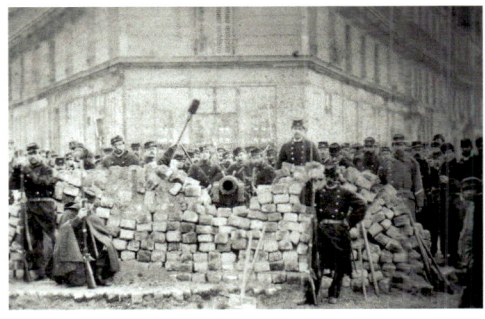

Paris Commune.

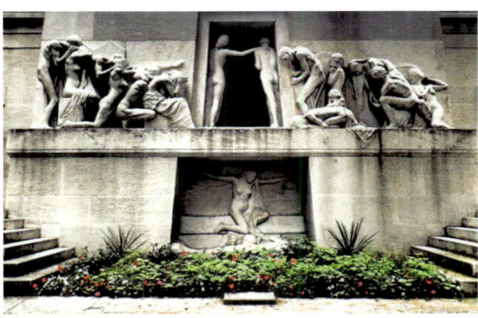

Père-Lachaise cemetery.

a communal grave. Eventually the government got the upper hand and the commune was short-lived. The death toll has been reckoned at just short of 7,000 government troops, and, of the Communards, an official count of nearly 900 but estimates of between 20,000 and 30,000, similar to or more than the number guillotined during the Revolution.

Adolphe Thiers (1797-1877)

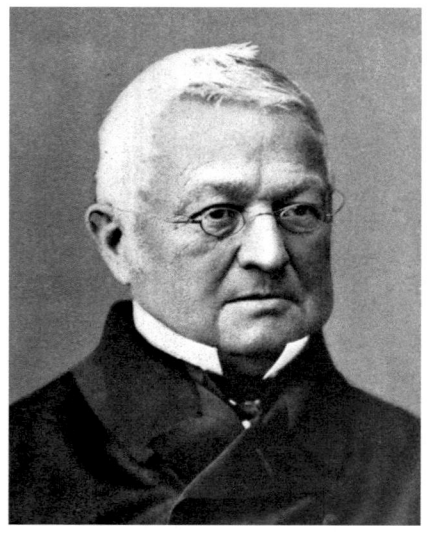

Adolphe Thiers.

Thiers was a highly influential figure in French history and perhaps should be better known than he is, whether as hero or villain can be debated. He was a left-leaning centre-ground figure occupying a place between the monarchist right and the more radical left. He was involved in the 1830 ousting of Charles X and was Prime Minister in 1836, 1840 and 1848. After the Franco-Prussian War he was chief executive of the government until August 1871 when he became President of the Third Republic.

He negotiated the settlement at the end of the war which was inevitable, though humiliating, and he ordered the military put down of the Commune. During his presidency he paid off the enormous debt owed to Germany and got rid of the last vestiges of German occupation. He had previously had the remains of Napoleon returned to Paris in 1840. Attacked on both sides by monarchists and left wing republicans he resigned in 1873 and died in 1877 at the age of 80. His funeral procession was led by two famous radicals, one more famous than the other, Victor Hugo and Leon Gambetta. Somewhere in his busy life he found time to write two gigantic tomes for which he received literary honours; a 10-volume history of the French Revolution and a 21-volume history of the Napoleonic consulate and empire. He must have had minions.

Georges Clemenceau (1841-1929)

Clemenceau was Prime Minister of France from 1906 to 1909 and again from 1917 to 1920. He qualified in medicine in 1865 and practiced medicine

12. The Paris Commune of 1871

in France and in the USA. He was a left winger but capable of fighting against the far left. During the Commune he was on the side of the Communards and for years after that he campaigned for an amnesty for them. He probably met Charcot at the home of Alphonse Daudet, and through his newspaper *La Justice* he supported Babinski in the row over his *aggregation* exams. He was a strong supporter of both Dreyfus and Zola and spoke eloquently at Zola's trials. At the Versailles conference after the First World War he demanded strong recriminations against Germany and secured the return of Alsace and Lorraine to France; no doubt he had vivid memories of the 1870 siege and the end of empire. He had been a strong opponent of Napoleon III. He was involved in the Panama Canal controversy which did for his reputation what involvement in the Parliamentary Expenses scandal of 2009 did for some MPs. He survived an assassination attempt in 1919 and he once fought a 'pretend' duel in which both fired three times and nobody was hurt.

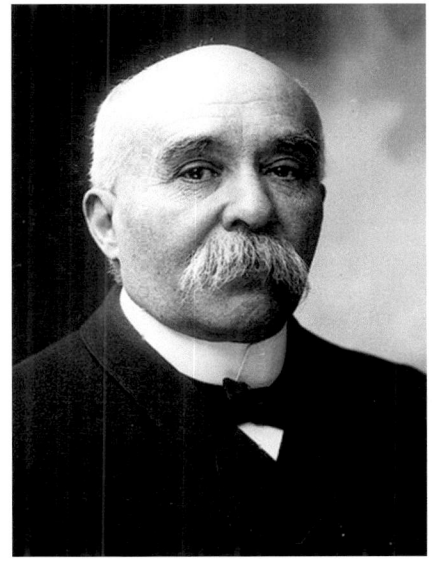

Georges Clemenceau.

Chapter 13

The Belle Époque (1871-1914)

Like the Edwardian era in Britain, the Parisian *Belle Époque* is looked on as a period of style and lightheartedness, especially for the upper classes. In France there were cultural, artistic, engineering and scientific advances and it was looked back upon with some relish compared with what followed in 1914 and after. Its beginning is ill defined and various sources give varying dates for it but all are agreed that it ended in 1914. Like the American historian Mary McAuliffe, I shall take it as starting after the end of the Commune.

Just thinking of the *Belle Époque* (the Good Times) is still capable of lightening the gloom even now after 150 years (or 107 years from the end of it). It wasn't all good, of course, and it's perhaps easier to label years good, or

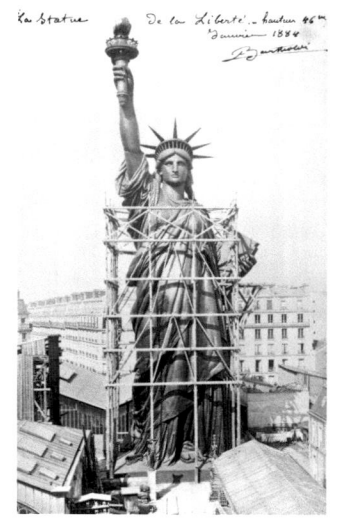
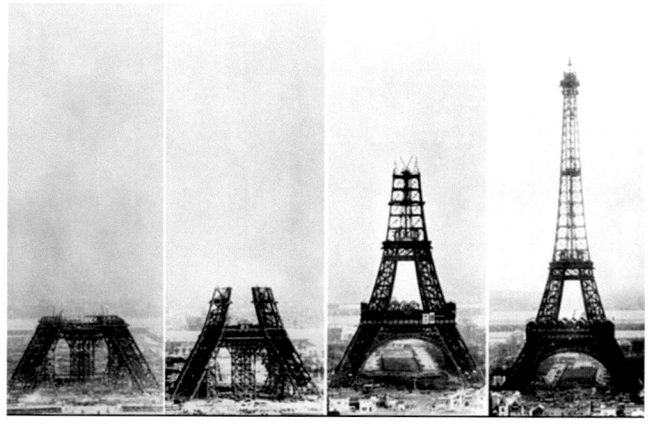

Above: Building the Eiffel Tower.
Left: Building the Statue of Liberty.

13. The Belle Époque (1871-1914)

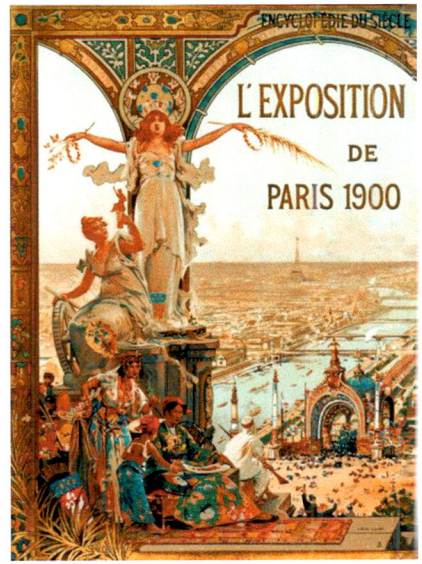

Paris Exposition.

beautiful, in retrospect than when you're living through them, especially for the deprived sectors of society, but to borrow a phrase from the 44th president of the United States, there does seem to have been a 'yes, we can' attitude and yes, they did. They built the Eiffel Tower, then the highest structure in the world; they built the enormous Statue of Liberty and shipped it to New York and they revolutionised (if that's not too loaded a word in French history) art, literature, music and popular entertainment. They had successful World Expositions in 1878, 1889 (the centenary of the revolution) and 1900. The Opera Garnier was built over a period of 14 years ending in 1875 by the architect Charles Garnier in Napoleon III style and became known as the Palais Garnier because of its extravagance, with its magnificent staircase, added to by Chagall with his beautiful ceiling painted in 1963 when he was 76. It's mainly used now for the ballet.

Impressionism got its name, intended cynically, from the painting *Impression Sunrise* by Claude Monet of the port of Le Havre in the hazy early morning light, first shown at the first impressionist exhibition held in 1874 after the traditional Paris Salon had spurned their work. That exhibition was joined by Renoir, Pissarro, Sisley, Cézanne, Morisot and Degas. Édouard Manet stayed away, he was staying loyal to the salon. Berthe Morisot was one of the impressionists but she had to overcome much sexual prejudice to become recognised as a talented member of the group alongside the men. She had a long friendship with Manet but married his brother Eugene.

Cézanne was the subject of something I knew quite firmly but quite wrongly for many years. I 'knew' that he had a habit of painting Mont Ventoux, so named because of the wind up there, especially when the Mistral blows when it can reach hurricane levels so that you might find yourself taking an unplanned flight. The mountain Cézanne was obsessed with, like Monet with his water lilies, was Mount Sainte Victoire, much smaller than Mt. Ventoux but nearer to his home

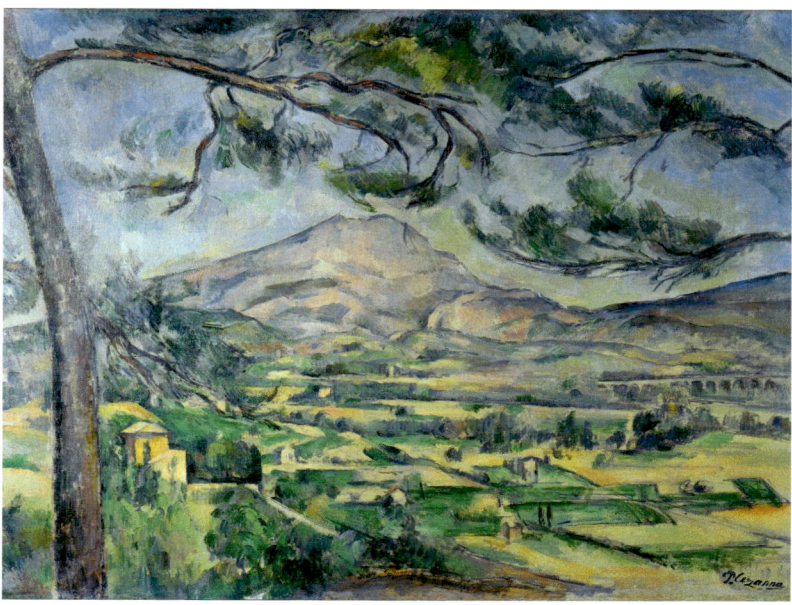

Mont Sainte Victoire with Large Pine *by Paul Cézanne.*

in Aix en Provence. In Aix (pronounced Aiks because of the ancient local language) you can't avoid Cézanne, who was a native, just as in Arles you can't avoid Van Gogh who was attracted there by the sun and the light, not that you would wish to avoid either of them in either place. Van Gogh died in 1890 and became the most famous of the post-impressionists in the decade after his death. We always intended to visit Giverny north west of Paris to see Monet's garden with its water lilies and the rustic arched wooden Japanese bridge but it was one

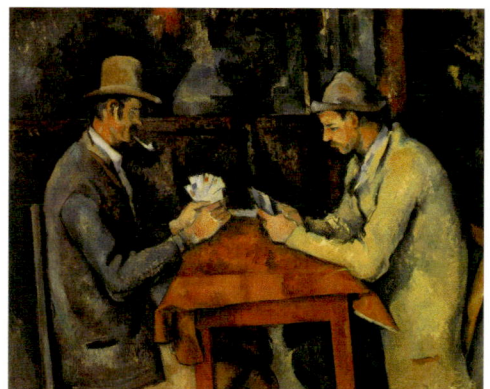

The Card Players *by Paul Cézanne.*

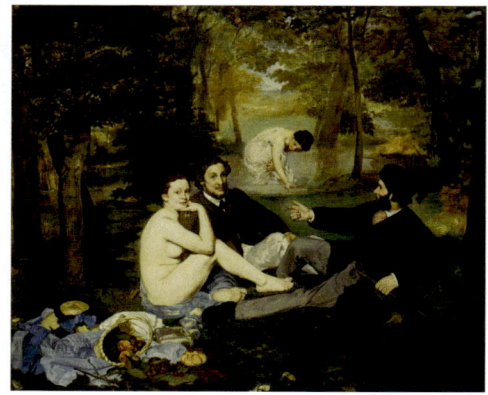

Le Déjeuner sur l'Herbe *by Édouard Manet.*

13. The Belle Époque (1871-1914)

of those things that never happened (on reading this my daughter has said we'll go together), Japanese art was an inspiration for the impressionists. Manet was abused because of his painting *Le Déjeuner sur l'Herbe* now regarded as a masterpiece but then considered beyond the pale because it portrays a naked woman between two fully clad men. The complaint then was about the naked woman; today it might be about inequality because the men aren't similarly undressed, but it doesn't seem clear why the woman had taken off her clothes in what otherwise seems to be a perfectly normal riverside picnic, unless it was a successful attempt by Manet to stimulate controversy. The woman was one of Manet's regular models, her name was Victorine Meurent. There has long been debate about whether Manet intended to represent her as a prostitute. With just a little stretching, Meurent can be read as dying (mourir; third person plural, present tense, *elles meurent*). OK, I know it should be *mourant*, but it's near enough to allow of a few flights of fancy; it shouldn't be a hindrance to the connoisseurs of dippiness. There must be some deep, unfathomable significance to it, of course. Victorine Meurent, victory before dying, glorious victory, death with the last shot of the battle, the theorising could be as endless as it would be pointless, like thinking that a woman must be for sale because she hasn't got any clothes on. Victorine was more than a model, she was herself an accomplished artist who exhibited at the Paris Salon and on one occasion her work was accepted when Manet's was rejected.

The age of art nouveau was short, from 1890 to 1910, but with its long flowing lines its remaining buildings are still impressive. I know there are some fine examples in Brussels. Perhaps its most striking example is the eye-smacking, Basilica of the Sagrada Familia by the Spanish architect Antonio Gaudi in Barcelona. Gauguin and Toulouse-Lautrec are said to be artists of the art nouveau, as is the Scottish designer, Charles Rennie Mackintosh. Mary McAuliffe tells a story of the actress Sarah Bernhardt (the divine Sarah) being stuck one Christmas for a poster for her current play, and she wanted it 'pronto' and she was very famous and very

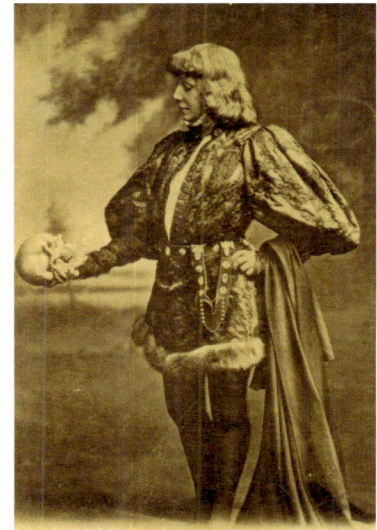

Sarch Bernhardt as Hamlet.

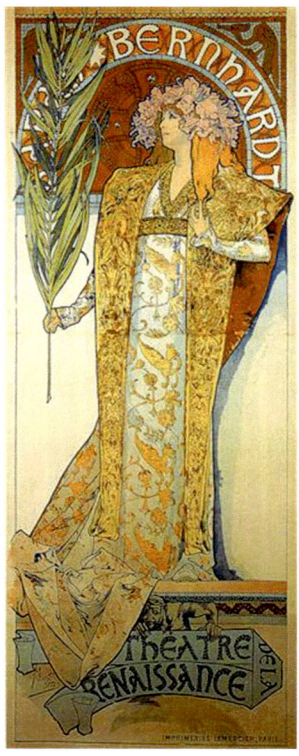

Sarah Bernhardt poster by Alphonse Mucha.

rich. The only artist to be found was a struggling Czech painter called Alphonse Mucha. He produced a poster that impressed her and was a hit in the fashionable circles of Paris. He hit the jackpot by producing for her, not only posters but much of the rest of her artistic needs, including her stage sets, her costumes and even her hairstyles. He became known as an artist of the art nouveau and beyond before returning to his native land.

Émile Zola (1840-1902) became famous and rich after the publication of his novel *L'Assommoir* (The Stunner) in 1877. He wrote his famous *J'Accuse* (the title was suggested by Clemenceau) open letter to the President in 1898, vehemently defending Captain Alfred Dreyfus. Dreyfus, who was Jewish, had been convicted of spying for the Germans and was given a life sentence and sent to the penal colony on Devil's Island in French Guiana. The 'Dreyfus affair' had divided France more surely, and much more poisonously, than Brexit divided Britain before and after 2016. It became an extremely bitter fight between, on the one side rampant and open anti-semitism and the so called honour of the French army, and on the other side the 'Dreyfusards', including an army of intellectuals such as Clemenceau, Anatole France, Marcel Proust, Monet and Sarah Bernhardt, who all believed in Dreyfus's innocence. For having the temerity to defend Dreyfus, Zola was convicted of libel against the army, twice, and given a prison sentence, but he fled to England and died in 1902 of carbon monoxide poisoning. Some have suggested it was a chimney-blocking murder. Six years after he was buried in a French cemetery, his remains were exhumed and placed in the Pantheon in Paris alongside those of Victor Hugo and Alexandre Dumas.

In 1906 the French High Court exonerated Dreyfus; he returned to army duties as Major Dreyfus and was given the *Légion d'Honneur*. The evidence against him had been fabricated. The army's top brass had been lying and cheating all along and prepared to see an innocent man fester, and probably

13. The Belle Époque (1871-1914)

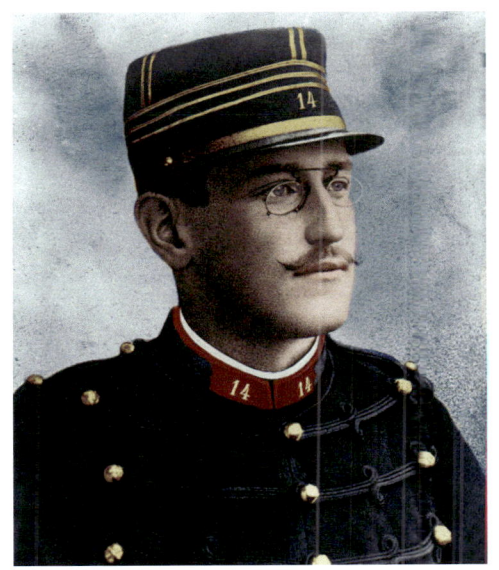

Alfred Dreyfus.

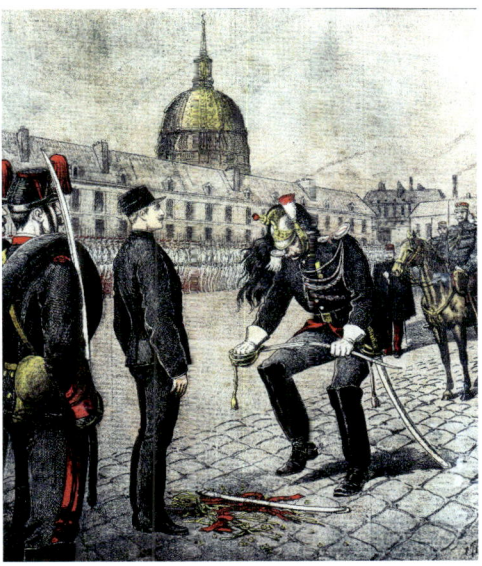

Decommissioning of Dreyfus.

die, on Devil's Island. It changed attitudes to wrongful conviction forever and Zola was recognised as a hero, a man who had everything but had risked it all to save a man he believed innocent. And he may, in the end, have paid for it with his own life.

Claude Debussy has often been spoken of as an Impressionist composer. He recoiled from the idea, saying that the application of the

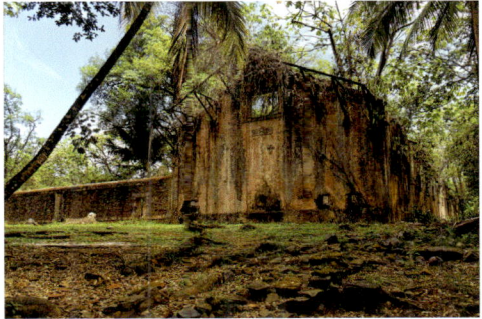

Devil's Island.

word 'impressionist' to either art or music was imbecilic. Others have said that his liking for themes of nature (*Claire de lune, L'aprés-midi d'un faune*) was similar to the '*plein air*' inclinations of the artists. The early reception of his music was similar to that afforded the works of the artists, but his favourite artist was Turner, who died in 1851.

Debussy (1862-1918) showed extreme musical talent at an early age and was admitted to the Paris Conservatoire at the age of ten. His father, Manuel, had been a supporter of the Commune and was imprisoned for his sympathies.

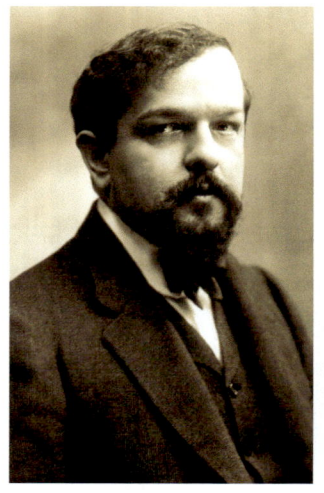 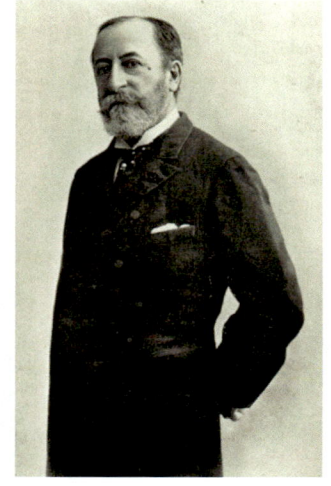 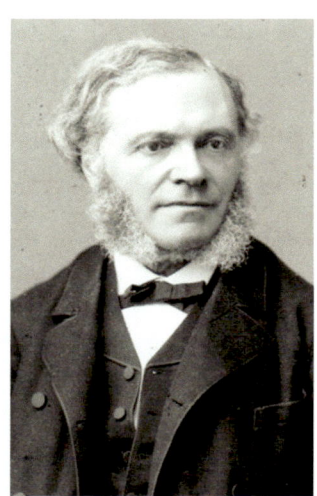

Claude Debussy. *Camille Saint-Saëns.* *César Franck.*

Debussy won the prestigious Prix de Rome in 1884 and that took him to the Villa Medici in Rome for further tuition but he hated it. His first success was his opera *Pélleas et Mélisande*, written in 1894, which brought him fame in 1902. In 1871 a group of composers led by Camille Saint-Saëns, and including César Franck and Jules Massenet had established the *Société National de Musique* in Paris. Other composers of the Belle Époque era included Stravinsky, Ravel, de Falla, Strauss, Respighi and Fauré. In 1872 Georges Bizet

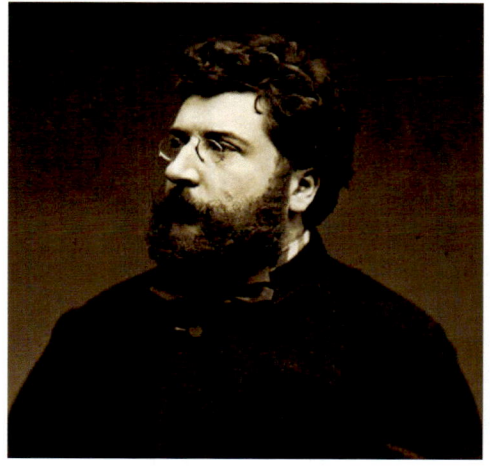 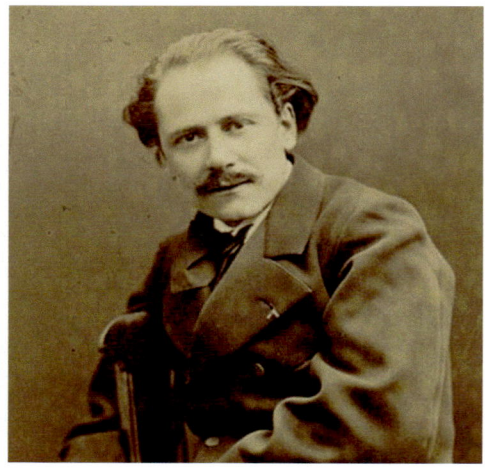

Georges Bizet. *Jules Massenet.*

13. The Belle Époque (1871-1914)

was commissioned by the *Opera Comique* to write an opera based on the novel, or novella, *Carmen* by Prosper Mérimée. Of course, it was panned by the critics after its first performance in 1875 before going on to become an accepted part of the operatic repertoire. Debussy was also a close friend of Erik Satie.

Apart from the Eiffel Tower, Cabaret is the most evident part of the *Belle Époque* that still persists in Paris especially the Moulin Rouge and the Folies Bergère. The Moulin Rouge was first opened in 1899 when it quickly developed a reputation as a disreputable sort of place, half cabaret and half brothel. It was burnt down in 1915 and rebuilt in time to reopen in 1921 after which it was revived by the dancer Mistinguett (it's respectable now). The can-can was developed from the quadrille in the early 19th century. Made famous by the Paris cabarets later in the century it was regarded by officialdom as improper and by the public as 'naughty but nice'. Performers such as La Goulue and Jane Avril, Charcot's long time patient, made it an essential part of the show.

In 2021 the Moulin Rouge (if you were allowed to go) would set you back £87.81 for the show and £166.84 if you opted for a meal with it. Whichever option you chose you would get champagne. The Folies Bergère predates the Moulin Rouge, having opened in 1869. It was originally built as an Opera House but soon 'changed its tune'. Manet's *A Bar at the Folies Bergère* was

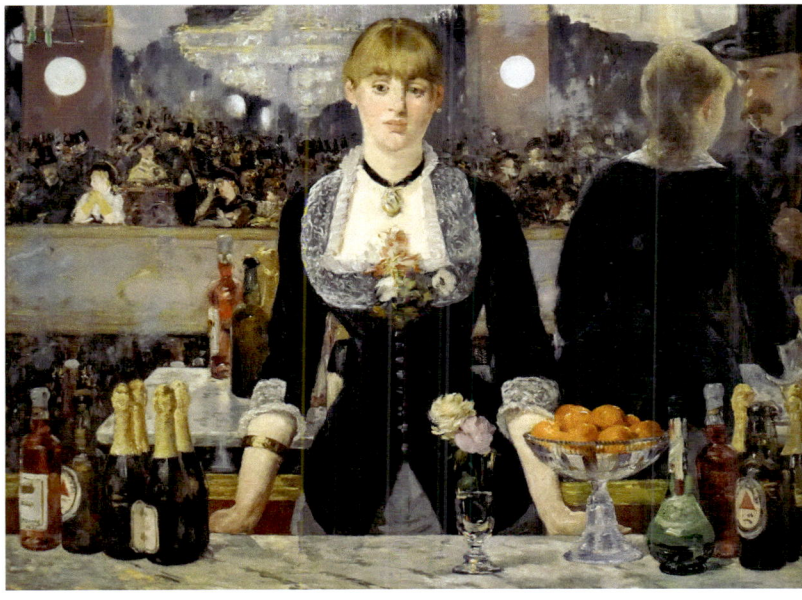

Manet's A Bar at the Folies Bergère.

painted in 1882, with its perfectly wholesome-looking barmaid in front of the bar mirror in which you can see the customers or patrons. 'A glass of white wine and a G and T please'. Performers would often work at both venues and past stars have included Charlie Chaplin, Maurice Chevalier, Charles Aznavour, Ginger Rogers, Edith Piaff, Ella Fitzgerald, Frank Sinatra and Elton John. The current price for the show (no meal) is 40 to 80 euros (£35-£70).

The great artist of the Cabaret, of course, was Toulouse-Lautrec, just as Degas was the great artist of the ballet and the racecourse. What was the cause of Toulouse Lautrec's shortness? My diagnosis would have been osteogenesis imperfecta (brittle bone disease) but it seems that he had another inherited bone disease called pycnodysostosis, sometimes now known as Toulouse Lautrec's disease or syndrome; the causative gene mutation is now known and can be tested for. He was too fond of the drink and, like Manet, Van Gogh, Alphonse Daudet and no doubt many others, he caught syphilis presumably in the Parisian nightlife of which he was so fond (it is disputed that Van Gogh had syphilis but he was treated for gonorrhoea). Towards the end of his life Toulouse Lautrec's mother had him committed to an asylum so perhaps he too had GPI or alcoholism, or both. He died at the age of 37. If you're ever driving past his hometown of Albi, not far to the northeast of Toulouse, (Toulouse Airport is fairly convenient for Provence) do stop and see the Toulouse-Lautrec museum.

The *Sacré Coeur* basilica began as an idea in the mind of the Archbishop of Paris in 1871 after the end of the Commune. The plan was that it should be a penance to God for the sins of the Revolution and of the Commune, so it was to be built on the site where the horrors of the 'bloody week' began. As you might imagine, that was the cause of a prolonged and monstrous argy-bargy between the secularists, including most of those who had supported the Commune, and the Catholics. The basilica's stone laying ceremony was

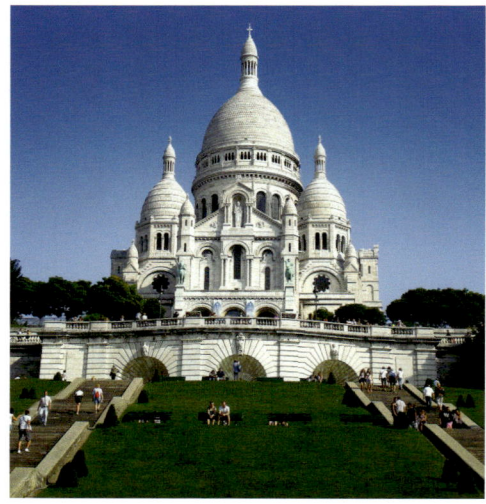

The Sacré Coeur.

13. The Belle Époque (1871-1914)

in 1875; it was finally consecrated in 1919. I have no religious affiliations, but it can't be denied that the *Sacré Coeur*, in its majestic whiteness at the top of the hill of Montmartre, is one of the finer sights of Paris and, indeed, of the world, a sort of French Taj Mahal without the romantic history of Shah Jahan and his uxorious devotion to his favourite wife, Mumtaz.

Our favourite spot in Paris was the *Place du Tertre* (the Square on the Hill), with its artists and its bustling atmosphere and the *Sacré Coeur* in the background, honeymoon perfection (artist offering to sketch Jennifer "Oh, my hair's a mess", "Mais madame, je vous coiffe"). The tiny things we remember clearly for the rest of our lives when we have forgotten so much else. I don't know whether I could ever go back to the *Place du Tertre* now and maintain my composure, even thinking about it has a strange effect; so many, so poignant memories. She was taken from us by cancer in 2014.

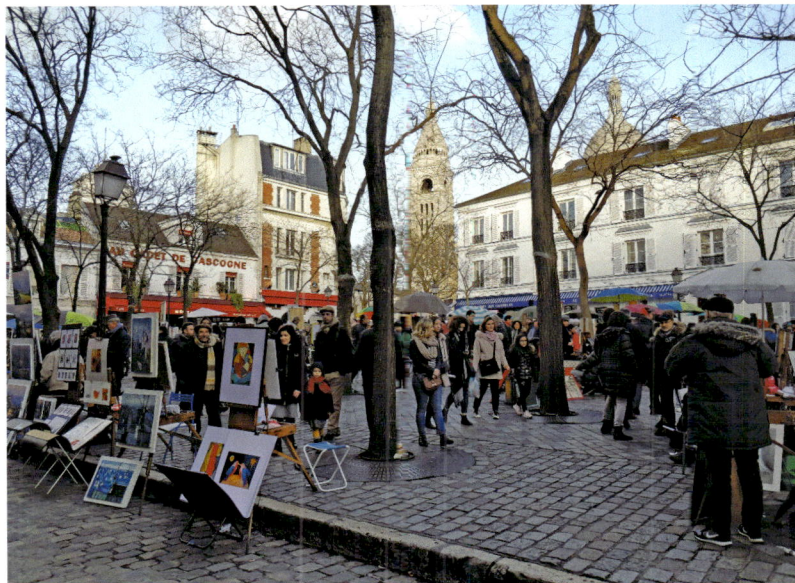

Place du Tertre.

Epilogue

The Salpêtrière Hospital began with despotism and tyranny; it descended even further to mass murder and sheer horror. But with the introduction of kindness and caring it was able to recover and, with the beginnings of psychiatry and neurology, became recognised as one of the leading hospitals of the world. It is now a busy general teaching hospital housing the medical school of France's most famous university, the Sorbonne.

Le Phénix est vraiment né des flammes.

On the 31st of August 1997, the world's most glamourous and popular Princess was involved in a car accident in a Paris tunnel. Diana was taken to the Salpêtrière Hospital where she died a few hours later at the age of 36. There was intense national mourning in her home country.

"Anywhere I see suffering, that is where I want to be, doing what I can."
Diana, Princess of Wales.

Bibliography

Erwin H Ackerknecht. *Medicine at the Paris Hospital, 1794-1848*. Johns Hopkins, Baltimore, 1967.

Michael Bliss. *Harvey Cushing: A Life in Surgery*. Oxford, New York, 2005.

Rutger Bregman. *Human kind: A Hopeful History*. Bloomsbury, London, 2021.

Matthew Cobb. *The Idea of the Brain*. Profile. London, 2020.

Macdonald Critchley, Eileen Critchley. *John Hughlings Jackson: Father of English Neurology*. Oxford, New York, 1998.

Harvey Cushing. *The Life of Sir William Osler – Vols. 1 and 2*. Oxford, New York, 1940.

Georges Didi-Huberman. *Invention of Hysteria* (Translated by Alisa Hartz). MIT Press. Cambridge, Massachusetts, 2003.

John F Fulton. *Harvey Cushing – A Biography*. Blackwell. Springfield, Illinois, 1946.

Christopher G Goetz, Michel Bonduelle and Toby Gelfand. *Charcot Constructing Neurology*. Oxford. Oxford, 1995.

Andrew Graham-Dixon. *Art, The Definitive Visual Guide*. Dorling Kindersley. London, 2008.

Georges Guillian. *J. M Charcot 1825-1893 – His Life His Work*. Hoeber. New York, 1959.

A McGehee Harvey. *Research and Discovery in Medicine*. Johns Hopkins. Baltimore, 1981.

Arthur Hassall. *Cardinal Mazarin*. Ozymandias. 2016.

Claire Joyes. *Claude Monet, Life at Giverny*. Thames and Hudson. London, 1985.

Michel Laclotte, Edward Lucie-Smith. *Impressionist Masterpieces at the Jeu de Paume, Paris*. Thames and Hudson. London, 1984.

Jeffrey A. Lieberman with Ogi Ogas. *Shrinks: The Untold Story of Psychiatry*. Weidenfeld & Nicolson. London, 2015.

Anthony Levi. *Louis XIV*. Constable. London, 2014.

Mary McAuliffe. *Dawn of the Belle Époque*. Rowman and Littlefield. Lanham, Maryland, 2014.

Peter Medawar. *Pluto's Republic*. Oxford. London, 1984.

William Osler. *Aequinimitas and other addresses*. HK Lewis. London, 1905.

Philippe Pinel. *Medico-Philosophical Treatise on Mental Alienation,* 1809 (Translated by Gordon Hickish, David Healy and Louis C. Charland). Wiley-Blackwell. Chichester, 2008.

Jaques Philipon, Jacques Poirier. *Joseph Babinski – A Biography*. Oxford. New York, 2009.

Roger Price. *A Concise History of France – 3rd edition*. Cambridge, 2014.

Mary M Robertson, Simon Baron-Cohen. *Tourette Syndrome – The Facts (2nd Edition)*. Oxford. Oxford, 1998.

Simon Schama. *Citizens – A Chronicle of the French Revolution*. Penguin. London, 2004.

Sue Bartolucci, Pat Forbis. *Stedman's Medical Eponyms – Second Edition*. Lippincott Williams and Wilkins. Baltimore, 2005.

Olivier Walusinski. *Georges Gilles de la Tourette: Beyond the Eponym*. Oxford. New York, 2019.

Index

Abbaye prison 15
acromegaly and pituitary tumour 65-6
Adrian, Edgar 95
Aicardi, Jean François Marie 68-70
Albutt, Clifford 43
Alzheimer, Alois 83-4
anaesthesia 85-6
Anne, Queen *4*, 5, 6
aphasia and dysphasia 57, 76, 78-9
appendicectomy 86
Archives de Physiologie 75
art nouveau 111-12
Avril, Jane 39

Babinski, Henri 53-4
Babinski, Joseph Jules François Félix 31, *32*, 37-8, 48, 68
    Babinski's sign 57, 59-60
    death 58-9
    early life and training 53-5
    and neurosurgery 57-8
Barré, Jean Alexandre 67, 68
beggars 4
Belle Époque 103-17
Bernard, Claude 72, 90-92
Bernhardt, Sarah 111-12
Bicêtre men's hospital 8, 15, 63
    boys' unit 43, 44
    psychiatric facilities 18
Biological Society of Paris (*La Société de Biologie de Paris*) 41-2, 57, 75
Bizet, Georges *114*, 114-15
bone disease 116

Bottard, Marguerite 33-4, 104
Bouchard, Charles 35, 52, 54-5
Bourneville, Désiré-Magloire 30, 31, *32*, 43-4
brain function 60, 76, 82, 84, 86, 95
breath holding 38
Bregman, Rutger 70
Brides of la Baleine 10-11
Brissaud, Édouard 31, *32*, 34, 40, 61-2
Broca, Paul Pierre 25, 75-6
Brouillard, Jean-Baptiste 76
Brown Institution, London 82, 95
Brown-Séquard, Charles Édouard 74-5, 78
Bruant, Libéral 7

Cabaret, the 115-16
Cajal Institute 82
cardiology 42, 79, 91
Casquette Girls 11
Cézanne, Paul 109-10
Charcot-Marie-Tooth disease *ix*, 66
Charcot, Jean-Baptiste-Étienne-Auguste 31, *32*, 44-6
Charcot, Jean-Martin 28, 30 *32*, 45-6, 54, 75-6, 93
    early life and training 28-30
    eponyms 35
    hysteria and 31, 37-9
    lecturing and teaching 31-3, 35, 48, 51-2, 61
    and Marguerite Bottard 33-4
    neurological conditions and 36-7

non-neurological diseases and 34-5
physical therapies 40
private and social life 40-42, 55-6
statue 41, *41*
Charité Hôpital 67
Charles X 101-3, 106
children *see* paediatrics
cholera 78
Chomel, Auguste François *xii*
chromosomes 27
Clemenceau, Georges 106-7
Commune (1871) 53, 105-6, 107
composers of the Belle Époque 113-15
Corday, Charlotte 15
Critchley, Macdonald 47, 79
Curie, Marie 39
Cushing, Harvey 84-9, 95

Daguerre, Louis 25
Dampierre, Marquise de 51
Dandy, Walter 87
Darwin, Charles 25
Daudet, Léon 46, 55
de Martel, Thierry 58, *59*, 83
Debussy, Claude 113-15, *114*
Decker, Auguste 84
Dejerine-Klumpke, Augusta Marie 63-4
Dejerine, Joseph 63, 66
Delasiauve, Louis 43
Diana, Princess of Wales 118
digestive function 91
Donné, Alfred François 25
Dreyfus, Alfred 107, 112-13, *113*
Duchenne type muscular dystrophy (DMD) 26, 80
Duchenne, Guillaume-Benjamin-Amand 23-7, 35, 41, 43, 50, 56
  death and memorial 26, 26-7, 56
  electrical apparatus 25, *25*
  muscle biopsy needle 26, *26*
Dupuytren, Guillaume 23-4

dysarthria 57
dysphasia and aphasia 57, 76, 78-9

ear mechanism 68
Eiffel Tower *108*
electrophysiology 25
endocrinology 65, 75
Enquist, Per Olav 39
epilepsy 37, 44, 69, 76, 78
Erb, Wilhelm Heinrich 25
Esquirol, Jean-Étienne Dominique 10, 21-3
eye treatment 78

Flexner, Abraham 85
Folies Bergère 115-16
France, Anatole 112
Franco-Prussian War 33, 53, 105, 106
French governance (1814-1940) 98-103
  Paris Commune (1871) 53, 105-6, 107
French Revolution (1789) 12-16, 98
French Revolution (1830) 10, 102-3
Freud, Sigmund 31, 37, 48
Fronde civil wars 4, 5

Gambetta, Leon 106
Garrod, Alfred Baring 34
general paralysis of the insane 50-51
Gilles de la Tourette, Georges Albert Édouard Brutus 31, *32*, 46-52
  after murder attempt (1893) 49-50
  Tourette syndrome 51-2
goitre 65
Golgi, Camillo 82
Goltz, Friedrich 95
gout 34-5, 39
Goutières, Françoise 69
Gowers, William Richard 79-81, 82, 83, 84

Index

Graves' disease 65
Guillain-Barré syndrome 67, 88
Guillain, Georges 37, 52, 66-8, 69

haemoglobin 80
Halstead, William Stewart 85-7
Heberden, William 52
Hertz, Cornelius 40
Hôpital des Enfants Malades 48
Horsley, Victor Alexander Haden 58, 65, 82-3, 86, 93, 95
Hôtel-Dieu 91
Hughlings Jackson, John 77-9
Hugo, Jeanne 46
Hugo, Victor 106
Hutchinson, Jonathon 77
hysteria 31, 37-9

impressionists and post-impressionists 109-111

Jenner, William 80
Johns Hopkins Hospital, Baltimore 85-6
    Hunterian Laboratory for Experimental Medicine 86-7
Johnson, Dr. Samuel 51

Kamper, Rose 49
Klumpke, Augusta Marie 63-4
Koch, Robert 93
Kocher, Theodor 86
Kraepelin, Emil 84

L-DOPA (levodopa) 19
Laennec, Rene *xii*, 23, 35, 50
Le Mécanisme de la Physionomie Humaine 25
Leborgne, Louis 76
les filles du roi 10
Levi, Anthony 3

Liberty leading the People 102, 103
Lieberman, Jeffrey 48
London Metropolitan Hospital 66
Louis Napoleon 91, 103-4, 107
Louis Philippe 103
Louis XIII 2, 4-5
Louis XIV 2-3, 5, 6, 7, 9, 10
Louis XVIII 100-101
lumbar puncture 79

Magendie, François 23-4, 91
Manandhar, Dharma *xi*
Manet, Édouard 109, *110*, 111
    A Bar at the Folies Bergère 115, 115-16
Manon Lescaut 8-9
Manual of Diseases of the Nervous System 80
Marat, Jacques-Louis 15
Marie, Pierre *ix*, 31, 32, 65-6, 76
Martel, Thierry de 58, 59, 83
Mazarin, Cardinal (1601-1661) 4-5, 6-7, 34
McAuliffe, Mary 108, 111
Medawar, Peter 48
medical exams system 56
medical schools 18, 20, 22-3, 29, 56, 77, 85
Medico-Philosophical Treatise on Mental Alienation 19
Mental Illnesses considered under the headings Medical, Hygienic and Medico-Legal 22
Meurent, Victorine 111
micro-organisms 92-3
Mills, Charles Karmer 34
Minkowski, Oskar 65
molecular asymmetry 92
Monet, Claude 109-10, 112
motor neurone disease 36-7
Moulin Rouge 39, 115

Mucha, Alphonse 112
multiple sclerosis 36
muscular dystrophy 26, 80

Napoleon Bonaparte 24, 100-101
Napoleon III 91, 103-4, 107
National Hospital, Queen Square,
    London 66, 75, 78, 80, 81, 83
Nelson, Horatio 23
neurophysiology 60, 83, 94-5
neurosurgery 57-8, 84
Nightingale, Florence *xii*
Nissl, Franz 83-4

obstetrics, 26, 27
Ochoa, Severo 82
ophthalmology 78
Osler, Grace 87
Osler, Revere 87-8
Osler, William 38, 39, 85, 88

paediatrics *ix*, 26, 27, 43-4, 63, 66, 68-70
Palais Garnier 109
palsy 25, 36, 63
Panama Scandal 40-41, 107
Paris Commune (1871) 53, 105-6, 107
Paris Faculty of Medicine 67
Parisian *Belle Époque* 103-17
Parkinson, James 36
Parkinson's disease 35-6, 39, 62
Pasteur, Louis 40, 56, 82, 85, 91, 92-4
Phipps, Alfred 80
photography, clinical 25
physiology 90-92
Pinel, Philippe 4, 17-21, 28, 40, 92
    and Esquirol 21-2
Pitié Hospital 56
pituitary 65-6, 87
Place du Tertre, Paris 117
Potain, Professor 56

prostitutes 7, 8-9
Proust, Marcel 57, 62, 112
psychiatry 17-21
    hysteria 31, 37-9
Pussin, Jean-Baptiste and Marguerite
    18, 19, *19*

Queen Square Nervous Diseases
    Hospital, London 66, 75, 78, 80,
    81, 83
Quincke, Heinrich Irenaeus 79

Ramón y Cajal, Santiago 81-2
Ramskill, J. Z. 78
Raymond, Fulgence 34, 62
Rayner, Professor P.F.O. 29-30
Revue Neurologique 62
Reynolds, John Russell 80
rheumatoid arthritis 34
Richelieu, Cardinal 4-5
Ringer, Sydney 38, 82, 86
Riva-Rocci, Scipione 86
Roberts, Dr. John *ix*
Robespierre 15-16
Roux, Émile 93

Sacks, Oliver 19
Sacré Coeur 116, 116-17
Saint-Saëns, Camille 114, *114*
St.Vincent de Paul 4, 5-6
Salpêtrière
    from arsenal to hospital 6-7
    building 7, *7*
        Babinski Building 57, *58*
        Pinel statue *21*
    Charcot's influence 30-31, 41
    A clinical lesson at the Salpêtrière 31-3, *32*, 38
    as detainment centre 8-10, 18
        deportations and emigrations 10-11

Diana, Princess of Wales 118
invasion of 'gilets jaunes' (2019) 71
patient called Marie 43-4
Pitié-Salpêtrière 56
professors of neurology (1894-1947) 61
psychiatric section and Marguerite Bottard 33-4
psychiatric treatment, early 18-21, 31, 37-9
Revolution (1789) and reign of terror 15
Schama, Simon 10
Sherrington, Charles 82, 86, 94-5
Snow, John 78
Société National de Musique 114
spinal hemisection syndrome 74-5
Statue of Liberty *108,* 109
Sydenham, Thomas 37
syphilis 39, 50, 116
syringomyelia 67

tabes dorsalis 35, 62, 67
Thatcher, Margaret 24
thermometry, clinical 43
Théroigne de Méricourt, Anne-Josèphe 9-10, 23
Thiers, Adolphe 106
Tooth, Howard Henry 66
Toulouse-Lautrec, Henri de 39, 116
Tourette, Gilles de la *see* Gilles de la Tourette
Tourette syndrome 51-2
Trousseau, Armand 25, 43

University College Hospital, London 83

vaccines 40, 80, 82, 93
Van Gogh, Vincent 50-51, 110
Victoria, Queen 27
Vincent de Paul 4, 5-6

Vincent, Clovis 58, *59*
von Helmholtz, Hermann 78
Vulpian, Edmé Félix Alfred 26, 36, 42, 63, 75

Walusinski, Olivier 46
wars 4, 5
Wittman, Marie (Blanche) 38
World Expositions, Paris 109, *109*

X-linked inheritance 27
X-rays 86

Zola, Émile 107, 112-13